Dryness, Tears, and Contact Lens Wear

CPCL
Clinical Practice in Contact Lenses

Series Editors

Gerald E. Lowther, O.D., Ph.D.
The Borish Center for Ophthalmic Research,
Indiana School of Optometry, Bloomington

Charles D. Leahy, O.D., M.S.
Assistant Clinical Professor of Optometry,
New England College of Optometry, Boston;
Contact Lens Service, Massachusetts Eye and
Ear Infirmary, Boston

Forthcoming titles:

Begley: *RGP Lens Fitting*
Zadnik and Barr: *Diagnosis, Fitting, and Care of the Keratoconus Patient*

Dryness, Tears, and Contact Lens Wear

Clinical Practice in Contact Lenses

Gerald E. Lowther, O.D., Ph.D.

The Borish Center for Ophthalmic Research,
Indiana University School of Optometry, Bloomington

Butterworth–Heinemann

Boston Oxford Johannesburg Melbourne New Delhi Singapore

Every effort has been made to ensure that the drug dosage schedules within this text are accurate and conform to standards accepted at time of publication. However, as treatment recommendations vary in the light of continuing research and clinical experience, the reader is advised to verify drug dosage schedules herein with information found on product information sheets. This is especially true in cases of new or infrequently used drugs.

Recognizing the importance of preserving what has been written, Butterworth–Heinemann prints its books on acid-free paper whenever possible.

Library of Congress Cataloging-in-Publication Data
Lowther, Gerald Eugene.
Dryness, tears, and contact lens wear / Gerald E. Lowther.
p. cm. -- (Clinical practice in contact lenses)
Includes bibliographical references and index.
ISBN 0-7506-9514-5
1. Contact lenses--Complications. 2. Dry eye syndromes.
I. Title. II. Series.
[DNLM: 1. Contact Lenses--adverse effects. 2. Dry Eye Syndromes--therapy. 3. Tears--secretion. WW 355 L922d 1997]
RE977.C6L684 1997
617.7'523--dc21
DNLM/DLC
for Library of Congress 96-39911
CIP

British Library Cataloguing-in-Publication Data
A catalogue record for this book is available from the British Library.

The publisher offers special discounts on bulk orders of this book.

For information, please contact:
Manager of Special Sales
Butterworth–Heinemann
313 Washington Street
Newton, MA 02158–1626
Tel: 617-928-2500
Fax: 617-928-2620

For information on all B–H medical publications available, contact our World Wide Web home page at: http://www.bh.com/med

10 9 8 7 6 5 4 3 2 1

Printed in the United States of America

To my wife, Andrya, and children, Karen and Daniel, for allowing me the many extra hours spent on this work and other professional activities while foregoing time that otherwise would have been spent in family activities

and

To my parents, Richard and Mary Alice Lowther, for the many years of unwavering support and encouragement

and

To the many colleagues who have made the observations, done the research, and published their results, which provide the background for a review like this to be written

Contents

Preface

This initial volume of the series on Clinical Practice in Contact Lenses covers the common contact lens problem of dry-eye symptoms with contact lens wear and other problems associated with tear film and contact lens wear. This in-depth discussion of the differential diagnosis and management of the marginal dry eye and related contact lens problems will allow the clinician to handle this very common clinical challenge.

The material is covered in a clinical problem-solving manner with sufficient background information for the reader to gain an in-depth understanding of conditions, mechanisms, and common management techniques. As with all clinical conditions, there are many manifestations of the same problem, and patients react differently to the same conditions and problems. One must understand the normal variation in test results and the need to do a battery of tests to determine the patient's problem and how to best treat it.

I would like to thank Victor Malinovsky and Carolyn Begley for their proofreading and suggestions for the manuscript.

Gerald E. Lowther

Dryness, Tears, and Contact Lens Wear

The Problem

Some of the most common problems with contact lens wear are related to the tear film. Twenty to thirty percent of patients using hydrogel lenses develop dry-eye symptoms when wearing their contact lenses. One survey of 214 patients wearing hydrogel lenses found that 21% of the male patients and 26% of the female patients had reduced wearing time attributable to dry-eye factors.[1]

Three hundred ten optometric and ophthalmologic practitioners who dispensed hydrogel contact lenses were surveyed concerning dryness symptoms and other wearing problems with the lenses.[2] One hundred sixty-two of these practitioners were randomly selected from around the United States; the remainder were selected from a dry climate (Arizona) and a humid climate (Washington state). They reported that 18–30% of their patients using hydrogel lenses had dry-eye symptoms; 12–21% had reduced wearing time because of these symptoms; and 6–9% could not wear contact lenses at all because of dryness symptoms. They ranked dry-eye symptoms as their third major problem (Table 1).

In another survey of 104 patients using hydrogel lenses, dryness was the most common symptom reported.[3] They were specifically asked if they (1) never, (2) seldom, or (3) often had the symptoms of scratchiness, dryness, or watery eyes. Figure 1 shows the percentage of patients with the various symptoms. When the patients were divided into male patients, women taking birth control pills, and women not taking birth control pills, it was found that the women taking birth control pills had a significantly higher frequency of dryness symptoms (Figure 2).

As is obvious from the above statistics, dryness symptoms are a major problem with hydrogel lens wear. Another problem associated with the tear film and lens wear is an increase in lens deposits with poor-quality tear film. The shorter the patient's tear film break-up time (BUT), the more rapidly deposits form.[4,5] Corneal staining can

Table 1. Ranking of the Most Important Problems with Hydrogel Contact Lenses Based on a Survey of Practitioners

Rank	*Problem*
1	Lens deposits
2	Lack of patient compliance
3	Dry-eye symptoms
4	Confusing care regimens
5	Ineffective lenses for presbyopia
6	Giant papillary conjunctivitis
7	Corneal physiologic changes
8	Insufficient lens parameters

Source: Modified with permission from GN Orsborn, SG Zantos. Practitioner survey: management of dry-eye symptoms in soft lens wearers. CL Spectrum 1989;4(9):23.

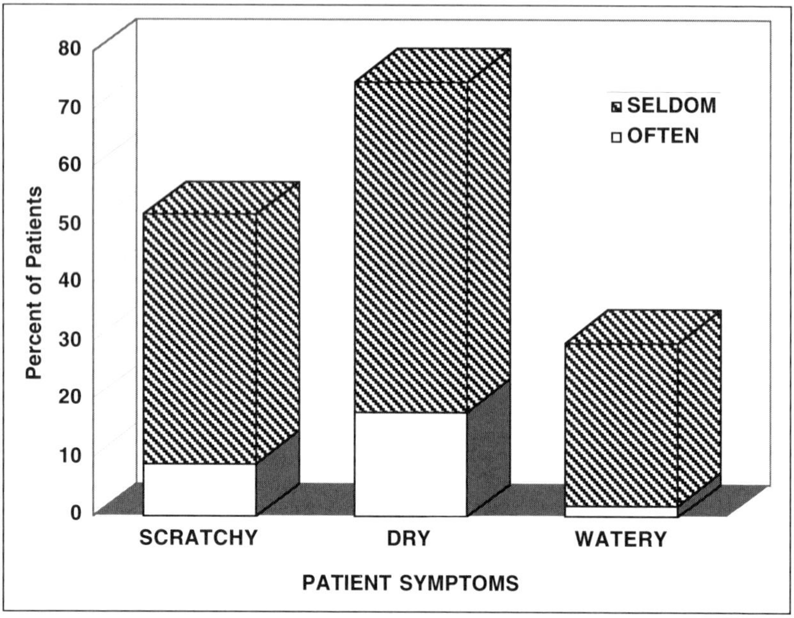

FIGURE 1. Percentage of patients wearing hydrogel lenses who indicate symptoms of scratchiness, dryness, and watering either often or seldom. (Modified from NA Brennan, N Efron. Symptomatology of HEMA contact lens wear. Optom Vis Sci 1989;66:834.)

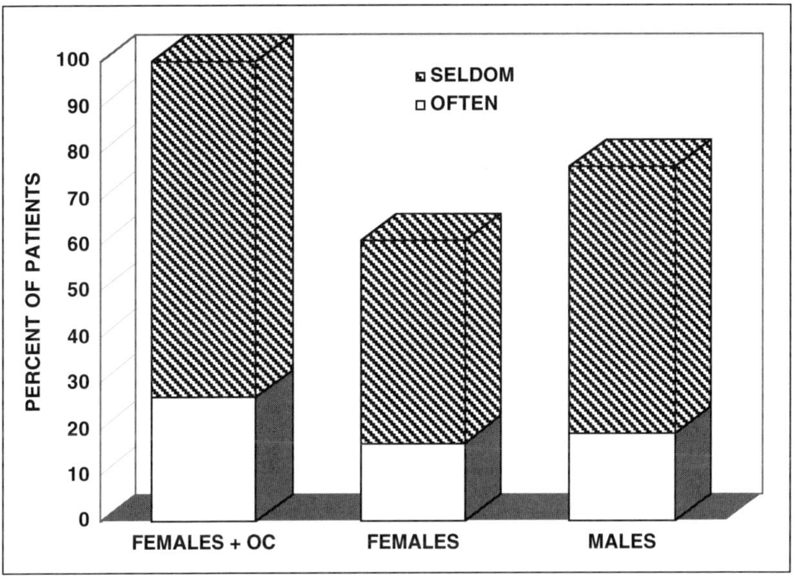

FIGURE 2. Comparison of the percentage of women taking oral contraceptives (OC), women not taking OCs, and male patients who have the symptom of dryness when wearing their hydrogel contact lenses. (Modified from NA Brennan, N Efron. Symptomatology of HEMA contact lens wear. Optom Vis Sci 1989;66:834.)

also be a result of hydrogel lens dehydration. With dehydration, hydrogel lenses tend to steepen, resulting in decreased movement and a tight fit. Hydrogel lenses will adhere to the eye during sleep, apparently because of the loss of aqueous tears under the lens. These and related clinical hydrogel contact lens–tear film interactions are explored in the following section.

There are also a number of adverse effects caused by tear film interactions with rigid gas-permeable (RGP) lenses. As with hydrogel lenses, the symptom of dryness is also a problem with these lenses; however, the incidence is not as high. There is the annoying surface debris-drying problem that affects patients' vision and comfort. Peripheral corneal staining (also called 3 and 9 o'clock staining, 4 and 8 o'clock staining, and peripheral desiccation) occurs to some degree in the majority of patients using RGP lenses. Adherence of the lens to the eye during sleep, and often for some time after awakening, occurs in 20–50% of the patients wearing lenses overnight and is related to the tear film. It occurs less commonly with daily wear. These problems with RGP lenses are explored in a later section.

Hydrogel Lenses and Tear Problems

Dehydration

In the early 1980s, Andrasko and Schoessler,[6] Andrasko,[7] Wechsler et al.,[8] and DeDonato[9] showed that lenses dehydrated while being worn.

Specifying Changes in the Amount of Water in a Lens

Hydration changes in hydrogel lenses have been defined in different ways. In other words, the same change in the amount of water in a lens may be reported as different percentages depending on the method used to calculate the change. There is no accepted standard method of reporting the change in water content of a lens and this has created confusion.

There are five ways of reporting the change in water content in a lens[10]:

1. Absolute change in lens mass

   $\Delta M = M - M'$

   where: ΔM is the change in mass

   M is the starting lens mass

   M' is the lens mass after the loss of water

   This is given in milligrams (mg).

2. Relative change in total lens mass

   $$\%\Delta M = \frac{\Delta M \times 100}{M}$$

   This is given as a percentage.

3. Relative change in lens water mass

$$\%\Delta m_w = \frac{\Delta m_w \times 100}{m_w}$$

Where Δm_w = change in the mass of the water in the lens

m_w = mass of the water in the lens

4. Absolute change in the lens water content

$\Delta W = W' - W$

Where $W = \frac{m_w \times 100}{M}$ and is the percentage of a lens by weight that is water.

This is given as a percentage.

5. Relative change in lens water content

$$\%\Delta W = \frac{\Delta W \times 100}{W}$$

The results from these different methods give quite different values as indicated in Table 2.

The water content of hydrogel lenses decreases very rapidly once placed on the eye. The greatest change in water content occurs within the first 5–10 minutes.[7,11] The amount of water loss is related to the thickness of the lens: The thicker the lens, the lower the percentage of water loss (Figure 3). This is most likely because the water is being lost from the anterior lens surface, with the lens dehydrating a given distance in from the surface before an equilibrium is established. If the anterior 0.05 mm of the lens is where the majority of the water is lost, and if the lens is only 0.05 mm thick, then it will lose a high percentage of water. On the other hand, if the lens is 0.10 mm thick, the percentage of water lost will be lower, even if the

Table 2. Different Values for the Amount of Water Loss Depending on the Method of Calculation

Definition	*38% Lens*	*75% Lens*
Absolute change in total mass	0.5 mg	12.1 mg
Relative change in total mass	3.1%	24.2%
Relative change in lens water mass	8.2%	32.3%
Absolute change in lens water content	2.0%	8.0%
Relative change in lens water content	5.3%	10.7%

Source: Modified from NA Brennan, N Efron, VT Truong, RD Watkins. Definitions for hydration changes of hydrogel lenses. Ophthalmic Physiol Opt 1986;6:333.

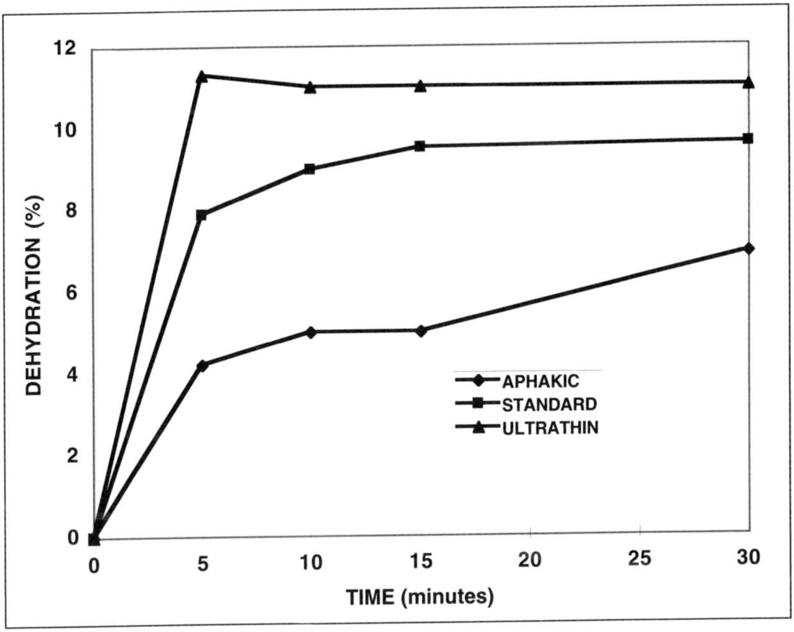

FIGURE 3. Rate of dehydration of hydrogel lenses of three different thicknesses (aphakic 0.51 mm; standard 0.13 mm; ultrathin 0.07 mm) on the eye. (Modified from G Andrasko. The amount and time course of soft contact lens dehydration. J Am Optom Assoc 1982;53:207.)

total amount of water lost from the two lenses is the same. It is important to understand this concept, as it may explain many of the clinical findings.

Decrease in Oxygen Transmission with a Decrease in Water Content

One of the adverse effects of dehydration of a hydrogel lens is that the oxygen transmission through the lens also decreases. The oxygen permeability of present hydrogel lens materials is exponentially related to the water content[12] (Figure 4). As the water content decreases, less oxygen is transmitted through the lens.

Paugh measured the change in oxygen uptake of the cornea with fully hydrated hydrogel lenses on as well as when the lenses dehydrated with wear.[13] He found that a fully hydrated 44.8% water content lens dehydrated to 37.1%. The equivalent oxygen percentage (EOP) decreased from 4.19% to 2.39%, which is a 57% drop in the amount of oxygen reaching the cornea. With no lens on the eye, the EOP would be about 21%, and if no oxygen reached the cornea it would be 0%. Using the relationship developed by Sarver et al.,[12] the oxygen permeability would be an equivalent of about 3.87% for the fully hydrated lens and 2.22% for the partially dehydrated lens, giving a 57% drop. Therefore, the decrease in oxygen permeability with on-eye dehydration could significantly increase corneal edema.

Part of the initial water loss when a fully hydrated lens is placed on the eye may be a result of the change in temperature.[14] Room temperature is approximately 20°C, whereas the ocular surface temperature is approximately 35°C. Table 3 shows the percentage of water lost as the temperature increases.

The starting water content of the lens is also important. In general, the higher the initial water content, the higher the amount of water that is lost with wear.[15] For example, a 73% water content lens will lose more water than a 38.6% water content lens (Figure 5). This is because there is more water in the surface layer to be lost; thus the

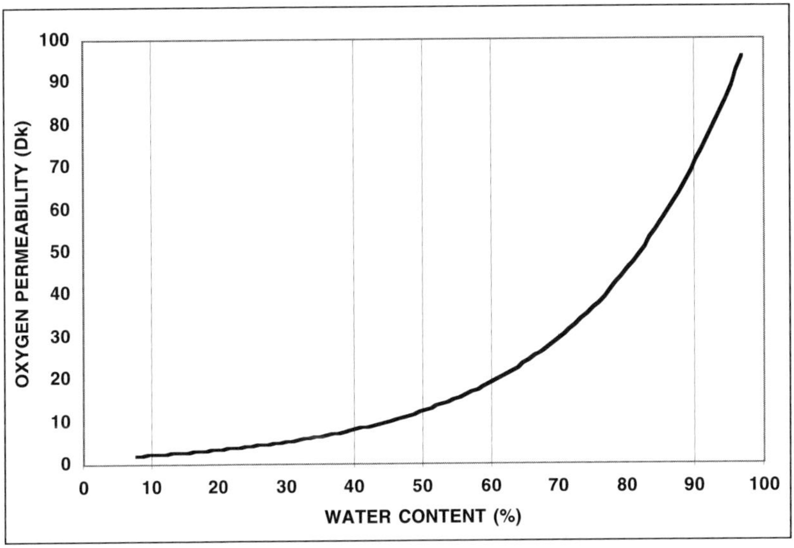

FIGURE 4. Relationship of oxygen permeability (Dk) to water content of hydrogel lens materials. (Data from MD Sarver, DA Baggett, MG Harris, K Louie. Corneal edema with hydrogel lenses and eye closure: effect of oxygen transmissibility. Am J Optom Physiol Opt 1981;58:386.)

Table 3. Lens Hydration Given as a Percentage of the Hydration at 20°C

Lens	*20°C*	*36°C*	*45°C*
Hydrocurve II (55%)	100	93.8	91.4
B&L 70 (70%)	100	89.6	86.1
Permalens (71%)	100	90.2	82.7

Source: Data from JE Kohler, GW Flanagan. Clinical dehydration of extended wear lenses. ICLC 1985;12:152.

amount of water lost from two lenses of equal thickness will be greater for the lens with the higher water content.

Environmental conditions can also affect the hydration level of lenses. Lower humidity conditions can cause a greater loss of water[15] (Figure 6). One study found no consistent correlation between low humidity and water content of hydrogel lenses; however, the humidity levels were relatively high, from about 40% to 90%.[16] The dehy-

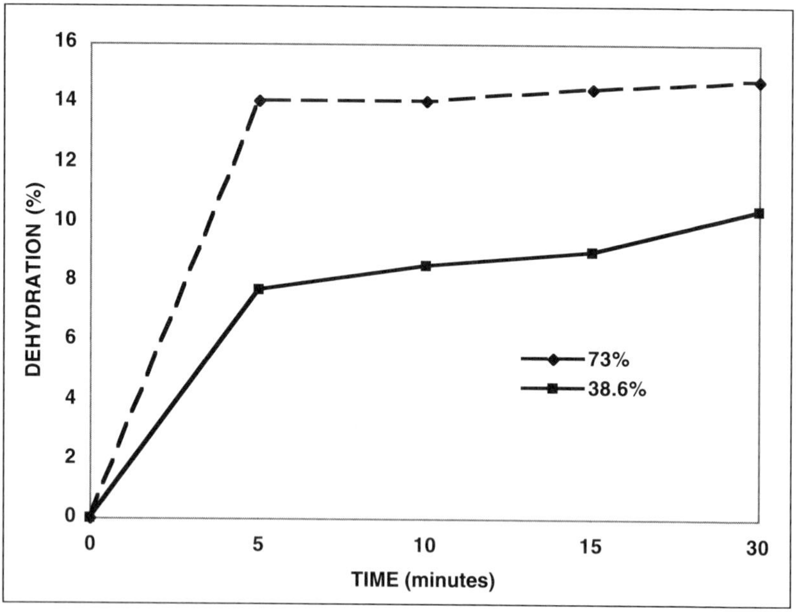

FIGURE 5. Effect of water content on the dehydration of hydrogel lenses. The higher water content lens loses more water. (Modified from G Andrasko. Hydrogel dehydration in various environments. ICLC 1983;10:22.)

dration problems appear to occur below 30% relative humidity. Another study[5] examined patients wearing hydrogel lenses who worked in environments with relative humidities varying from 15% to 48%. Using a scale of 0–3 for discomfort, the investigators found that patients in humidities less than 31% had the greatest discomfort (Figure 7). The tear film BUT on the lens surface was shorter for those in the low humidity work places as well

Low humidity is an important factor in many climates and under numerous other conditions. For example, in colder climates in the winter with a heating system with no humidifier, the relative humidity can go below 20%. In arid climates the humidity is often 20% or less. During commercial airline travel, many contact lens patients complain of dryness symptoms; this is most likely a result of the low humidity in the airliner cabin, which may be 15% or less.

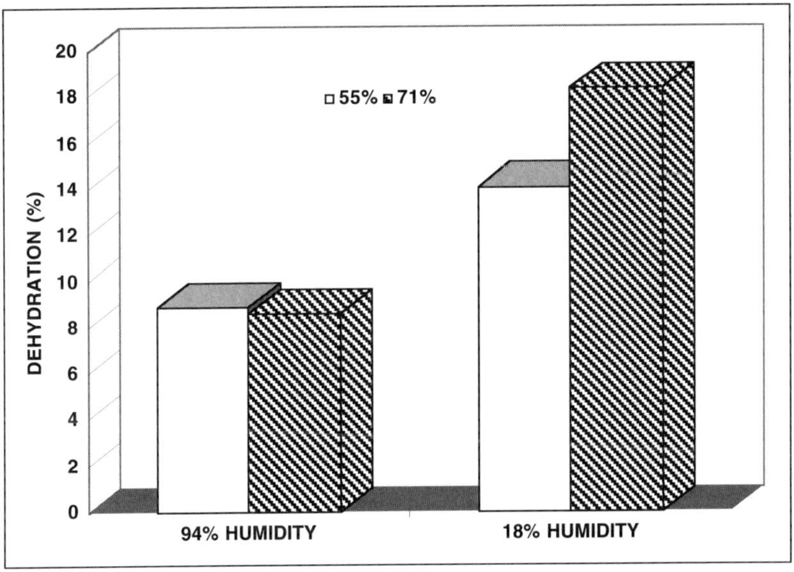

FIGURE 6. In high humidity conditions there is less water lost from a hydrogel lens than at low levels of humidity. (Modified from G Andrasko. Hydrogel dehydration in various environments. ICLC 1983;10:22.).

Windy conditions can also accelerate dehydration, thus increasing symptoms.[15] Patients working under or near heating or cooling ducts that increase air flow or patients in windy environments may have greater problems.

The presence and thickness of the lipid layer on the surface of the contact lens is important in retarding evaporation from the lens. It has been shown that the lipid layer is compromised on the surface of contact lenses. Guillon[17] has shown that rigid lenses essentially do not have a lipid layer, whereas the lipid layer is variable on hydrogel lenses. Korb[18] indicated that the lipid layer on hydrogel lenses is rarely similar to that on an eye not wearing a lens. He also found that the quality of the lipid layer was very dependent on the humidity. It was found that a high humidity (over 70%) was required to form a normal lipid layer on hydrogel lenses and in some cases a 100% humidity environment was required. Guillon[19] also found that lens

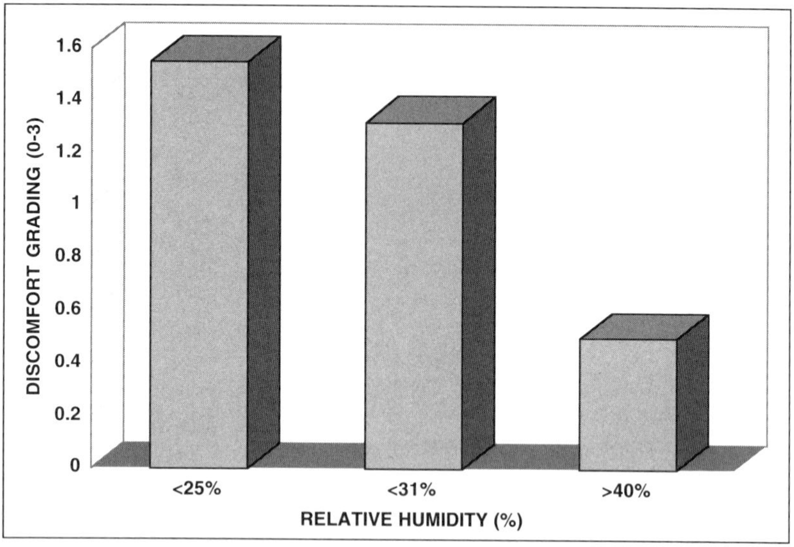

FIGURE 7. The grading of hydrogel lens discomfort (0, no discomfort, to 3, maximum discomfort) for patients in different relative humidity environments. (Data from SEG Nilsson, L Andersson. Contact lens wear in dry environments. Acta Ophthalmol 1986;64:221.)

thickness was a factor. A more normal lipid layer, thicker and more stable, was formed on thicker lenses (0.06 mm) than on thin lenses (0.035 mm). He also found that the lipid layer was thinner on high water content lenses than on lower water content hydroxyethylmethacrylate (HEMA) lenses.

Blinking is important in maintaining the lipid layer because it both forces the lipid from the meibomian glands and spreads it over the surface of the cornea or contact lens. The thickness of the lipid layer on the tear film of non–contact lens wearers varies considerably. Korb et al.[20] found it to vary from less than 60 nm to 180 nm in a group of 104 patients. Figure 8 shows the distribution of thicknesses. The thickness of the lipid layer can be estimated from the appearance of the interference fringes seen with white light and the biomicroscope. They are easiest to see in the inferior portion of the cornea using broad beam (4–5 mm wide) illumination. They can also be seen on the surface of contact lenses. With very thin

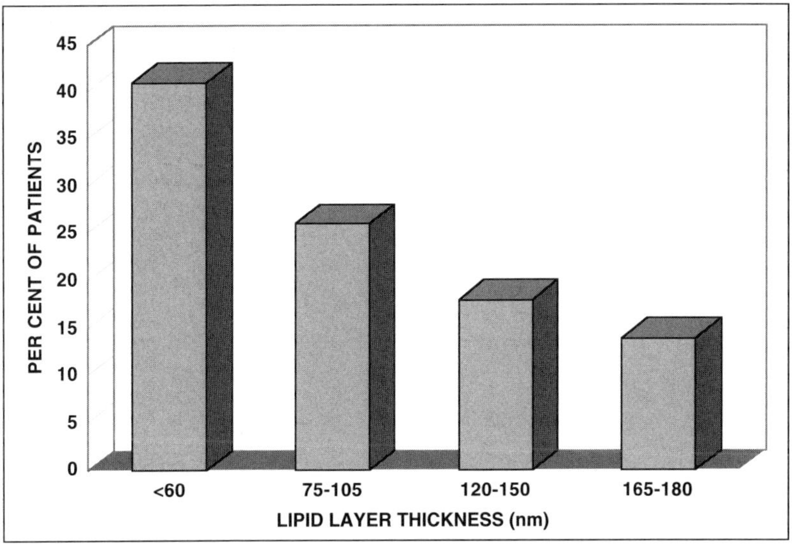

FIGURE 8. The lipid layer thickness of a sample of normal patients. (Data from DR Korb, JP Herman, JM Exford, et al. Tear film lipid layer thickness as a function of blinking. Cornea 1994;13:354.)

lipid layers no pattern will be seen; however, as the thickness of the lipid layer increases, the interference fringes become apparent. Table 4 gives the correlation of the thickness with the fringe color. The colors are easy to see after expression of the glands by light pressure on the lid margin or after a forcible blink. After three forceful blinks Korb et al. found an average increase in the lipid layer of 26 nm. When they compared subjects with thicker lipid layers (75–150 nm) with those with thinner lipid layers (<75 nm), the change in lipid layer thickness after the blinks was much less for those with initially thin lipid layers. Thus, it appears that the individuals with thin lipid layers who we would expect to have more drying problems also have less lipid secreted with forceful blinks.

Cedarstaff and Tomlinson[21] found that placing a soft contact lens on the eye caused a significant disruption of the tear film, resulting in a significant increase in evaporation of tears from the ocular surface. A disruption of the oily layer would give this result. They did

Table 4. Color of Interference Fringes and Corresponding Lipid Layer Thickness

Color	*Thickness (nm)*
Blue	180
Blue/brown	165
Brown/blue	150
Brown	135
Brown/yellow	120
Yellow/brown	105
Yellow	90
Gray/yellow	75
Gray	60
Gray/white	45
White	30

Source: Modified with permission from DR Korb, JP Herman, JM Exford, et al. Tear film lipid layer thickness as a function of blinking. Cornea 1994;13:354.

not find the increased evaporation to be consistently related to the initial water content of the lens.

A decrease in blink rate (longer interval between blinks) would increase the amount of dehydration of a lens. The blink rate is affected by a number of factors. It has been shown that low blink rates are associated with a high level of mental performance[22] and with increasing difficulty of the visual task.[23–26]

Practitioners who dispense contact lenses know that soft lens wearers who use video display terminals (VDTs) extensively complain of dryness symptoms. When using VDTs, patients tend to blink less.[27,28] Patel et al.[29] found a dramatic decrease in blink rate with VDT use (Figure 9).

Corneal sensation is important in initiating a blink. With corneal anesthesia the blink rate has been found to significantly decrease.[30] The decrease in blink rate with concentrated visual tasks such as reading, VDT use, or driving is probably made worse with the wearing of soft contact lenses because of the decrease in stimulation to blink. The presence of the lens decreases corneal sensation from air movement and drying. Thus, often the lens surface must dry to the point of caus-

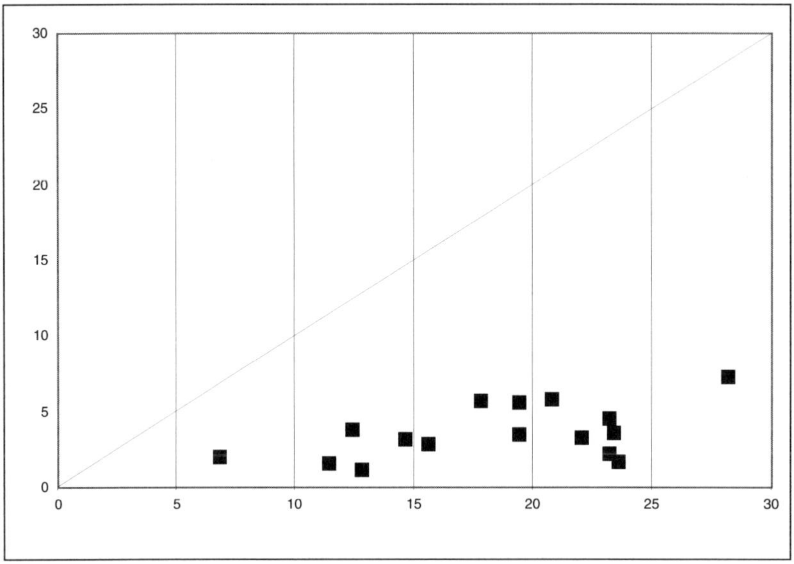

FIGURE 9. Comparison of the blink rate with video display terminal (VDT) use versus that during normal conversation. Note how all the points fall below the line indicating lower blink rates with VDT use. (Data from S Patel, R Henderson, L Bradley, et al. Effect of visual display unit use on blink rate and tear stability. Optom Vis Sci 1991;68:888.)

ing a decrease in vision before the patient blinks. However, one study found an increase in blink rate with soft lens wear after about 3 weeks of adaptation.[31] A recent study indicates that women using birth control pills have a significantly increased blink rate when compared with men or women not taking the medication.[32]

What We Know About Hydrogel Lens Dehydration

1. Thinner lenses lose a greater *percentage* of water.
2. Increased temperature decreases water content.
3. Higher water content lenses lose more water.
4. More water is lost under low humidity conditions.
5. Decreased blink rate increases lens dehydration.

Lens movement decreases with dehydration. Patients in lower humidity conditions with short lens surface BUTs showed less movement than patients in environments with higher humidity.[5] The mechanism may be that the lens tends to shrink and steepen, resulting in less movement. Other mechanisms such as a thinning of the tear film under the lens could also be the cause.

Corneal Staining

Dehydration of hydrogel lenses on the eye can cause corneal staining.[33–35] The fluorescein staining is characterized by punctate spots that often stain rather intensely (Plate 1). With the lens on the eye or before the instillation of fluorescein the spots appear white and flakelike (Plate 2). This staining usually occurs within the palpebral aperture.

Dehydration staining is worse with thin, high water content lenses and less with thick, low water content lenses. Figure 10 shows the effect of water content and thickness.[35] With lenses 0.04 mm thick and 70% water content worn for 4 hours, the staining was graded 1.5 on a 0–4 scale. The 0.04-mm–thick 38% water content lenses on the same patients (the high water content lens was placed on one eye and the low water content lens on the other eye) developed staining graded as 0.6. In a second study, when two 70% water content lenses with thicknesses of 0.14 mm and 0.05 mm were compared, the thin lenses resulted in 65% of the eyes having staining grades of 2–4 (significant) and 15% having grades 3 or 4. With the thick lenses, only 12% of the patients had grade 2 staining and no patients had grades 3 or 4. Lens movement (0.4 mm versus 1.2 mm) did not appear to effect the amount of staining.

The humidity will affect the amount of staining with thin, high water content lenses.[33–35] Figure 11 shows the change in corneal staining (scale 0–4) with wearing time for 75% water content lenses, 0.06 mm thick.[34] In this study the low humidity condition was a relative humidity of 53%, whereas the high humidity condition was

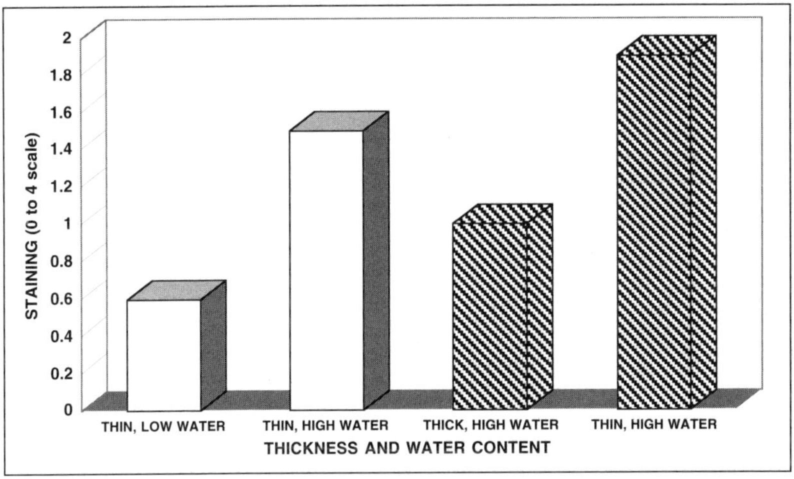

FIGURE 10. The effect of lens thickness and water content on the amount of corneal staining from dehydration. Open bars show one experiment with 0.04-mm–thick, 38% and 70% water content lenses. The cross-hatched bars show the effect of 0.05-mm and 0.14-mm–thick 70% water content lenses. (Data from GN Orsborn, SG Zantos. Corneal desiccation staining with thin high water content contact lenses. Contact Lens Assoc Ophthal J 1988;14:81.)

created by having the patient wear goggles that increased the humidity to 87%. This confirms dehydration as the cause.

The relatively common condition with hydrogel lens wear of arcuate staining[36] (also called "smile" staining) is, at least in some cases, caused by dehydration (Plate 3). It occurs in the most exposed area of the cornea that is least likely to be wiped by the lids and is the last area covered and first uncovered by the lids during a blink. Use of rewetting agents and thicker, low water content lenses may decrease or eliminate this staining.

Facts About Dehydration Staining

1. Greater with thinner lenses
2. Greater with high water content lenses
3. Worse in low humidity conditions
4. Usually occurs within the palpebral aperture

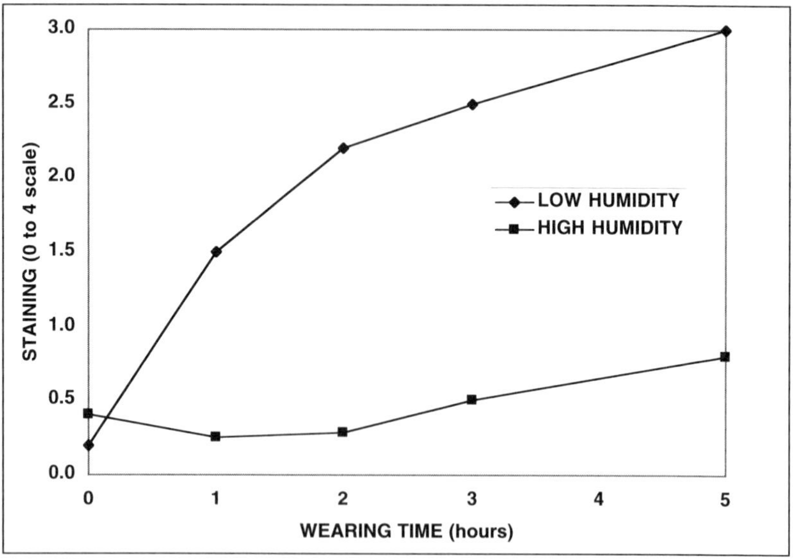

FIGURE 11. The amount of staining for 0.06-mm–thick, 75% water content lenses worn in a low humidity (53%) and high humidity (87%) environment. The greater staining is with low humidity. (Modified with permission from BA Holden, DF Sweeney, RG Seger. Epithelial erosions caused by thin high water content lenses. Clin Exp Optom 1986;69:103.)

Lens Adherence

If you were to wake a patient who was sleeping in the morning with a hydrogel lens on his or her eye and try to move the lens before the first blink, most likely you would find the lens stuck. This adherence is very common. One study has indicated an incidence of adherence of hydrogel lenses of 48% with overnight wear.[37] The lens will usually start to move after the first few blinks. The cause of the adherence is not fully understood. From what has been learned from the adherence of rigid lenses, it is expected that it is caused by a loss of the majority of the aqueous layer from under the lens with the remaining mucous layer acting as a glue.[38] The appearance of the tear layer under the lens supports the idea that there is little or no aqueous layer.[39]

The question is, "Why is the aqueous layer lost?" One reason may be that during sleep, the level of tearing greatly decreases. Apparently there is not a basal rate of tear production; tearing is caused by stimulation of the anterior surface of the eye from drying, air movement, and other disturbances. When a person is under general anesthesia, there is almost no tear production.[40] This stimulation also is not present during sleep. The lens may become somewhat drier or the tear fluid may become more hypertonic, and water is drawn from under the lens. When a stuck lens is removed, it feels drier and stiffer, as if it is dehydrated. One study did not find lenses to be dehydrated on awakening; however, in this study the lenses were removed and the water content measured by the patients using a refractometer.[41] Because the patients obviously had to have been awake for some time before the lenses were removed, there was sufficient time for the lenses to rehydrate, since the lenses start moving and seem hydrated after just a couple of blinks. Another factor may be that the lens may not move during sleep and the constant pressure of the lid forces fluid from under the lens.

The theory that the mucus plays a part is made more feasible by the recent findings that the mucoid layer may be much thicker than previously thought. It has been generally accepted that the tear film is about 6.5–7.5 μm thick, with the mucin layer a fraction of this.[42] However, Prydal et al.[43,44] have reported that the mucin layer alone may be 30–44 μm thick and previously was not measured as part of the tear film. The mucin layer is apparently soft and spongy or gel-like. Mucin is viscoelastic.[45] Thus, it is feasible that the lens may get pushed into this layer if the lens does not move for some time, resulting in adherence.

Clinically we might ask, “What difference does it make whether or not the lens moves during sleep?” Adherence could contribute in a number of ways to problems seen with extended wear. Bacteria may be trapped under the lens and held in place for long periods of time. Undisturbed under the lens with nutrients in this warm condition, the bacteria may multiply and have a chance to attack an area of damaged epithelium. The adherent lens will also trap waste products of corneal metabolism and epithelial cells sloughed off the corneal surface (Plate 4).[46] It has been shown that large numbers of epithelial and inflammatory cells (a mean of 119 epithelial cells and 6,500 leukocytes) are present in the eye after sleep, whereas a mean of only 7.5 epithelial cells and 9 leukocytes are seen during the open eye situation.[47] When a contact lens was worn overnight, the number of leukocytes were somewhat higher (8,154). Tan et al.[48] found similar cell counts with the overnight wear of hydrogel lenses. This trapped material may contribute to epithelial dysfunction and could be implicated in such conditions as microcyst formation and a decrease in epithelial adhesion. Decaying material trapped under the lens may cause an immune response. Lens adherence during sleep might also cause corneal trauma, giving opportunistic bacteria a site for infection. If the lens adheres to the epithelial cells, then on eye opening and blinking an area of epithelium may be pulled off. It has been shown that epithelial adhesion decreases with extended lens wear.[49] Areas of full-thickness epithelial defects resembling recurrent erosions have been seen with extended lens wear.[50]

Deposit Formation

Patients with short tear film BUTs have been shown to develop deposits at greater rates than those with long BUTs (Figure 12).[4] This probably occurs because when proteins dry, their conformation is lost and they are denatured. This is similar to what occurs when proteins are heated.

Patients working in low humidity conditions (<31%) have significantly greater levels of deposits than those working in higher humidities.[5] In the same study they confirmed the association of higher deposit levels with low BUTs.

Conjunctival Changes

A number of changes have been observed in the bulbar conjunctivae of hydrogel contact lens wearers. In one study all the asymptomatic soft contact lens patients studied showed evidence of squamous cell

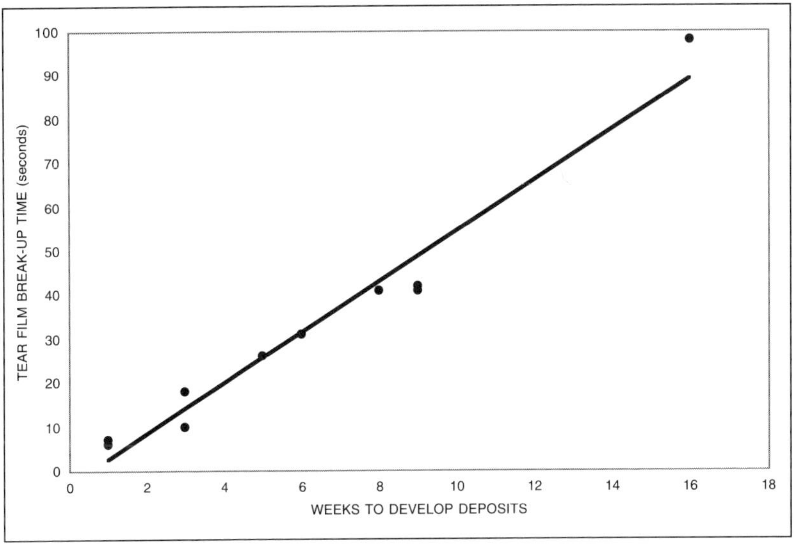

FIGURE 12. The correlation of the rate of deposit formation to the tear film break-up time. (Modified from RA Hathaway, GE Lowther. Factors influencing the rate of deposit formation on hydrophilic lenses. Aust J Optom 1978;61:92.)

metaplasia with enlarged, flattened cells but without keratinization.[51] The greatest changes were in the upper bulbar conjunctiva, where most of the cells were abnormal. The increase in cell size was the result of an increase in the cytoplasm of the cell and not the nucleus. In some cases the cell sizes were double normal size. There were elongated snakelike structures of nuclear chromatin in the conjunctival cells. They occurred most frequently in the upper bulbar conjunctiva with 25% of the cells showing the changes, although the changes were found in cells throughout the entire conjunctiva. Previously these cellular changes had only been observed in dry-eye patients and only in the upper conjunctiva. This raises the possibility that contact lenses cause changes in the conjunctiva similar to those that lead to the symptom of dryness in dry-eye patients. These cellular changes could be caused by mechanical effects, metabolic changes, or inflammation. The changes were found to be reversible with discontinuation of contact lens wear.

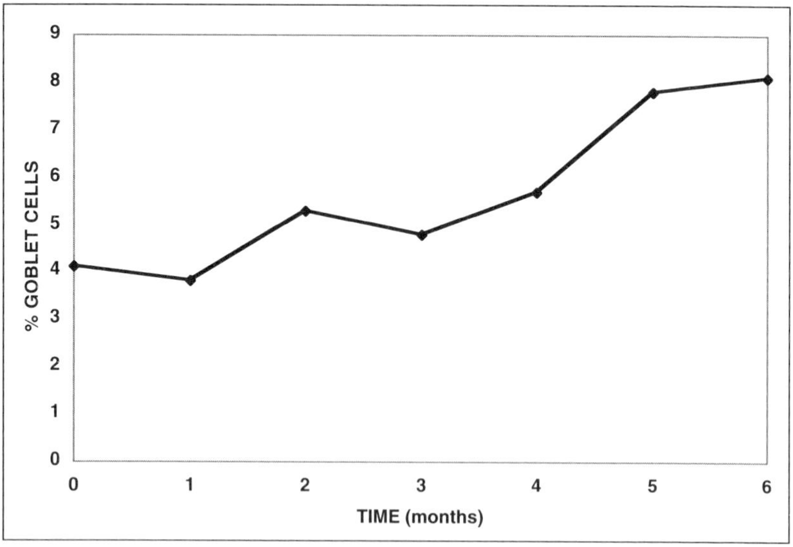

FIGURE 13. The increase in goblet cells in the conjunctiva with months of hydrogel lens wear. (Modified with permission from CG Connor, JB Campbell, SA Steel, JH Burke. The effects of daily wear contact lenses on goblet cell density. J Am Optom Assoc 1994;65:792.)

Another change that appears to occur with contact lens wear is a change in the number of goblet cells in the conjunctiva. Griener and Allansmith[52] showed an increase in the mucus-containing vesicles in contact lens wearers. Recently Connor et al.[53] showed a doubling of the number of goblet cells in the conjunctivae of new contact lens wearers over the first 6 months of lens wear (Figure 13). The percentage of goblet cells in the conjunctival samples as determined by impression cytology increased from 4.19% to 8.08%. An increase in goblet cells could increase the mucin production, further increasing deposits and lens adherence.

Examination of Patients and Predicting Tear Film–Related Problems with Hydrogel Lens Wear

We would like to be able to predict which patients wanting to wear contact lenses will develop the symptoms and problems associated with lens dehydration and ocular dryness. With such predictive powers we could either not fit some of these patients or use certain types of lenses, wearing schedules, lens care regimens, and dry-eye treatment programs to minimize the problems.

It is not always possible to predict which patients will develop significant problems with dryness symptoms before fitting them. However, we can identify those patients who have marginal dry-eye signs and symptoms before fitting them with lenses. Careful questioning and examination procedures are required.

Case History

The most important "test" in diagnosing a marginal dry-eye patient is the case history. Many patients will demonstrate only symptoms, often mild and elusive, and not have any objective signs.

The types of sensation reported by patients with dry eyes vary considerably. In a survey of practitioners in which they were asked to indicate the symptoms most commonly reported by dry-eye patients, a sandy, gritty feeling was reported by the greatest number (Table 5).[54]

In a group of 177 patients not wearing contact lenses, McMonnies and Ho reported that soreness followed by scratchiness were the most common symptoms.[55, 56] Of patients diagnosed with keratoconjunctivitis sicca, dryness and grittiness were the most common symptoms (Table 6).

Table 5. Most Common Symptoms in Dry-Eye Patients as Reported by Practitioners

Symptom	*Percentage*
Sandy, gritty feeling	92
Burning sensation	83
Red, irritated eyes	75
Excessive tearing	75
Stringy mucous discharge	40
Photophobia	37
Morning complaints	48
Stabbing pain	23

Source: Modified from FJ Holly. Diagnosis and treatment of dry eye syndrome. CL Spectrum 1989;4(7):37.

Table 6. Symptoms Reported by Patients with Keratoconjunctivitis Sicca Versus Normal Patients Reporting for an Ocular Examination*

Symptom	*Sicca*	*Normals*
Soreness	46%	24%
Scratchiness	32%	22%
Dryness	78%	19%
Grittiness	63%	14%
Burning	32%	3%

*Based on 37 normal subjects and 63 keratoconjunctivitis sicca patients—all women over 45 years of age.
Source: Data from CW McMonnies, A Ho. Patient history in screening for dry eye conditions. J Am Optom Assoc 1987;58:296.

Figure 14 is a questionnaire that can be used to determine if a patient has a dry-eye condition. Such a questionnaire can be used to identify contact lens candidates who might develop symptoms with contact lens wear or those who have a frank dry eye and should be discouraged from being fitted with contact lenses.

Medications can have a profound effect on the tear film and symptoms of dryness. Patients on certain medications will have problems with contact lens wear. Medications may also explain why a patient who has been wearing contact lenses without problems suddenly develops dryness symptoms. Patients must be carefully

DRY EYE QUESTIONNAIRE

Name: ______________________ Age: ______ Sex: M F Date: ____________

Occupation: ____________________________

Do you ever experience any of the following symptoms?

Symptom	**Frequency (check one)** never	sometimes	often	constantly
Sandy or gritty feeling				
Burning				
Dryness				
Soreness				
Scratchiness				
Itching				
Eye discomfort on awakening				
Tearing (watery eyes)				
Foreign body sensation				
Eye pain				
Redness				
Mucus discharge				
Light sensitivity				
Blurred vision				
Infections of the lids or eye				
Hayfever				
Other allergies				
Nasal congestion				
Cough				
Bronchitis				
Cold symptoms				
Sinus congestion				
Dryness of throat, mouth, or vagina				
Trouble swallowing food				
Asthma symptoms				
Joint pain				
Muscle pain				

Do your eyes seem overly sensitive to (circle all that apply):

cigarette smoke	swimming
smog	alcohol
air conditioning	sunshine
heaters and air blowers	wind
dust	use of video display terminals
pollen	

(continued)

FIGURE 14. Questionnaire used in the prefitting examination to determine if a patient has a dry eye.

Do you wear contact lenses?	yes	no
Have you previously tried to wear contact lenses?	yes	no
Do you use artificial tears or drops?	yes	no
Have you ever been told you sleep with your eyes open?	yes	no
Have you ever been treated for dry eyes?	yes	no
Do you take antihistamines?	yes	no
Are you taking birth control pills?	yes	no
Are you taking diuretics ("water pills")?	yes	no
Are you taking any other medications? (either prescribed or over-the-counter)	yes	no

If yes to above, give brand name and reason for taking: ______________________________

____

Have you or any blood relative had any of the following conditions (check all that apply and if a relative, indicate relationship):

Condition	**Yourself**	**Relative**	**Relationship**
Arthritis			
Thyroid disorder			
Lupus			
Sarcoidosis			
Asthma			
Sjögren's syndrome			
Skin disorders			
Heart disease			
High blood pressure			
Gout			
Cataracts			
Diabetes			
Glaucoma			

Other systemic conditions: ______________________________________

____

FIGURE 14. (continued)

Table 7. Medications That Can Affect the Tear Film and Cause Dry-Eye Symptoms

- Antibiotics
  - Tetracycline
- Antihistamines
  - Allergy medications
  - Sinus medications
  - Sleep medications
  - Diet medications
- Antihypertensives
  - Methyldopate hydrochloride
  - Reserpine
- Antiperspirants (long-term)
- Belladonna alkaloids
  - Bellergal
  - Donnatal
  - Pro-Banthine
- β-Blockers (topical)
- Birth control medications
- Botulinum toxin
- Dermatologic medications
  - Isotretinoin
- Diuretics
  - Chlorothiazides
  - Furosemide
  - Hydrochlorothiazide
- Psychotomimetics
  - Chlordiazepoxide
  - Diazepam
  - Amitriptyline
  - Thioridazine

questioned about any medications they may be taking. Be sure the patient reports not only medications prescribed to them but any over-the-counter medications they are taking. Some patients even do not consider birth control pills to be a medication. Table 7 gives some common medications that can cause dryness.

All patients reporting for an examination wearing contact lenses should be questioned about lens comfort and dryness. As was pointed out, a large percentage of patients with hydrogel lenses report dryness. The questions in Figure 15 can help determine if a patient is having drying problems with lens wear.[57]

With respect to the rapidity of the onset of dryness, one study of 35 hydrogel lens patients with dryness symptoms indicated that about 36% of the patients reported dryness symptoms within 1 hour of lens wear. In another 36% dryness first developed 1–3 hours after lens wear began, in 10% it developed between 3 and 5 hours after lens wear began, and in 18% of the patients the drying did not occur until they had worn their lenses at least 5 hours (Figure 16).[58]

Objective Testing

Examination of the Lids

The slit-lamp biomicroscope examination should start with a good evaluation of the lids and lid margins. Is there good apposition of the lids to the globe? Is there any trichiasis, entropian, or ectropian? Are there any deformities of the lid structure that prevent normal and total closure of the lids with a blink? Do the lids close completely with a blink? If with a blink the lids do not close completely, there will be more lens drying and corneal staining.

With dry eye there is commonly dried mucoid material along the lid margin. This is easiest to see after the instillation of fluorescein and by pulling the lower lid slightly away from the globe (Plate 5).

BLEPHARITIS. It is common to have blepharitis either alone or associated with meibomian gland dysfunction. Bowman et al. classified chronic blepharitis into six categories (Table 8).[59] The most common blepharitis with contact lens patients is staphylococcal blepharitis, which occurs because of the young age of most contact lens patients. Collarettes of material around the base of the lashes are an important diagnostic sign (Plate 6). There may also be scruf, dry scaly material, at the base of the lashes. The lid margin is commonly

CONTACT LENS PATIENT QUESTIONNAIRE

Name: ______________________________ Age: _____yrs. Sex: M F

How long have you worn contact lenses: _______yrs. _______mos.

How old are your present contact lenses?_______weeks or _______months

Do you use disposable or frequent replacement lenses? yes no

If yes, how often do you replace them? _______weeks

How many hours per day do you normally wear your contact lenses: _____hrs.
(if extended-wear answer 24 hrs.)

Do you ever experience any of the following eye symptoms while wearing your contact lenses? (circle all that apply)

soreness dryness grittiness burning no symptoms

If you have the above symptoms, on an average day how often do the symptoms occur? (circle one)

never sometimes often constantly

If you have the above symptoms, on an average day how many hours do you wear your contact lenses before these symptoms occur? (circle the one that applies)

less than 1 hour
1 to 3 hours
3 to 5 hours
greater than 5 hours

Do you use eye drops (rewetting, saline, artificial tears or other drops) while wearing your contact lenses? yes no

If yes, how many times per day?_______times

Do you regard your eyes as being unusually sensitive to cigarette smoke, smog, air conditioning or central heating? yes no

Do you have eye irritation as you awake from sleep?

never sometimes often every day

Do you experience dryness of the nose, mouth, throat, chest or vagina?

never sometimes often every day

Do you suffer from arthritis? yes no

Are you taking any medications (including over-the-counter and birth control pills)? yes no

If yes, list those you are taking. ______________________________

____

FIGURE 15. Questionnaire used to determine if a patient is having a problem with dryness with contact lens wear.

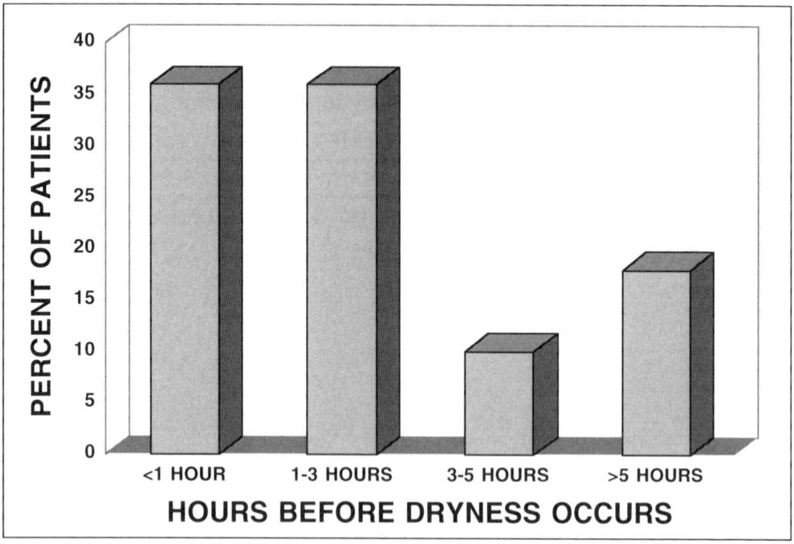

FIGURE 16. Time of lens wear before the symptom of dryness occurs for a group of 35 patients with dryness symptoms. (Data from TG Slusser. Effects of Lacrimal Drainage Occlusion with Non-Dissolvable Intracanalicular Plugs on Hydrogel Contact Lens Related Dry Eye. Master of Science Thesis, University of Alabama at Birmingham, 1994.)

Table 8. Classification of Blepharitis According to Bowman and Colleagues

Staphylococcal blepharitis
Seborrheic blepharitis
Pure seborrhea
With staphylococcal component
Meibomian seborrhea
Secondary meibomianitis
Primary meibomianitis

Source: Data from RW Bowman, JM Dougherty, JP McCulley. Chronic blepharitis and dry eyes. Int Ophthalmol Clin 1987;27:27.

inflamed and in severe cases can have an ulcerated appearance. The lid margins should be examined for hyperemia, thickening, and irregularity of the margin. Telangiectasia (an increase in the number and visibility of the blood vessels) is common with blepharitis, especially seborrheic blepharitis. With seborrheic blepharitis, the scaling

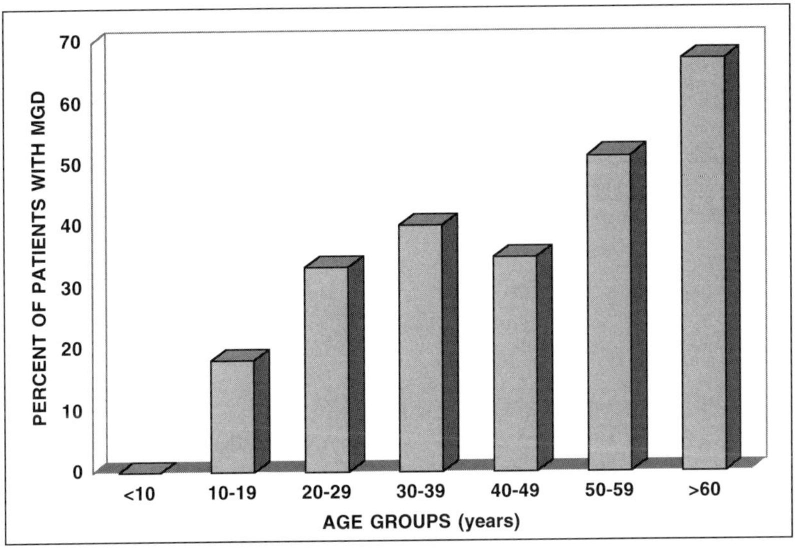

FIGURE 17. Percentage of patients from a randomly selected group of 398 patients reporting for a vision examination with meibomian gland dysfunction (MGD) at each age range. (Redrawn from MM Hom, JR Martinson, LL Knapp, JR Paugh. Prevalence of meibomian gland dysfunction. Optom Vis Sci 1990;67:710.)

may be more oily or greasy. There may be a loss of lashes (madarosis) or the lashes may be misdirected. There may be a chronic papillary conjunctivitis and an inferior keratitis (Plate 7) in the lower part of the cornea from staphylococcal toxins.

MEIBOMIAN GLAND DYSFUNCTION. Meibomian gland dysfunction is a common cause of dryness symptoms and is quite prevalent. In a study of 398 patients reporting for routine vision examinations, 38.9% were found to have meibomian gland dysfunction based on either a cloudy secretion on gland expression or an inability to express material.[60] The percentage of patients with meibomian gland dysfunction increases with age (Figure 17).

Korb and Henriquez compared 38 patients with contact lens intolerance with 40 contact lens patients with no symptoms.[61] In the symptomatic patients they found a higher incidence of foam along the lid margins and in the canthi and corneal staining after one

Table 9. Signs of Meibomian Gland Dysfunction in a Group of Symptomatic Contact Lens Patients Versus a Group of Contact Lens Wearers Without Symptoms

Patients	*Foam*	*Corneal Staining (1 instillation)*	*Corneal Staining (2 instillations)*
Symptomatic	66.2%	19.7%	57.7%
Control	3.7%	6.3%	10.0%

Source: Data from DR Korb, AS Henriquez. Meibomian gland dysfunction and contact lens intolerance. J Am Optom Assoc 1980;51:243.

Table 10. Percentage of Meibomian Glands From Which Oil Could Be Expressed with Mild Pressure

Patients	*All Glands Released Secretion*	*Some Glands Released Secretion*	*No Glands Released Secretion*
Symptomatic	9.9%	53.5%	36.6%
Control	57.5%	40.0%	2.5%

Source: Data from DR Korb, AS Henriquez. Meibomian gland dysfunction and contact lens intolerance. J Am Optom Assoc 1980;51:243.

instillation of fluorescein and after a second instillation (Table 9). Likewise, they found an increase in plugged glands (Table 10). The meibomian gland excretory ducts probably become blocked by epithelial cells because of increased turnover of these cells or abnormal keratinization. This blockage can result in stagnation of the secretion and bacterial infection.

Clinically, meibomian gland function can be evaluated with several techniques. One is to just view the openings of the glands along the lid margins. If the glands are normal, only small openings will be seen, with no pouting (a dome appearance of material coming out of the glands) or plugging present. As the degree of the dysfunction increases, the amount of pouting (Plate 8) and the number of plugged glands increases. Often fluorescein helps visualize the pouting of the glands.

The ease with which the lipid can be expressed from the glands is also an indication of the degree of dysfunction. With normal glands, mild pressure on the exterior of the lid just below the lashes will cause a clear liquid to be expressed from the glands. As the condition worsens, it is more difficult to express material from the glands. The expressed material becomes white or yellow in color. A plug of hard material may be forced out of the gland before any lipid is expressed. In severe cases it may be almost impossible to express the glands even with considerable pressure.

Foaming (bubbles) in the tear meniscus and at the canthus is a common sign of meibomian gland dysfunction, and the degree increases with the severity of the dysfunction. There may be an increase in debris in the tear film and meniscus. The tear film BUT decreases with increased severity of the dysfunction. It has been found that the tear film BUT for patients with meibomian gland dysfunction was greatly decreased (mean 7.18 seconds) and generally below 9 seconds, whereas control patients had a mean value of 28.22 seconds.[62] It was also found that with the re-establishment of the lipid layer after expression of the glands, the BUT returned to normal values.

Lid margin and conjunctival changes also occur. The conjunctiva becomes more injected and congested. There may be increased staining with rose bengal and an increase in palpebral hypertrophy. The lid margins become injected, swollen, and distorted.

The meibomian glands can also be viewed by transillumination. The lower lid can be everted over a standard transillumination source and then viewed with the low magnification of the biomicroscope. If the glands are normal, they will appear as straight lines. As the dysfunction increases they become more dilated, engorged, and irregular in shape. Collections of lipid may be seen, with "microchalazia" seen in more advanced cases. Patients with advanced dysfunction may develop chalazia.

Patients will report increased symptoms with advancing severity of the dysfunction. They may initially report mild foreign body sensation, irritation, tearing, burning, and dryness only with contact lens wear. As the condition worsens, these symptoms increase in severity, and they report crusting along the lid margins as well as increase redness of the lid margins. They may report a history of chalazion. This is a chronic condition, and thus patients may have a long history of these symptoms and even believe these are normal sensations.

In an excellent in-depth discussion of meibomian gland dysfunction, Caroline and Kame provided a 0–4 classification scale that is very useful in the clinical diagnosis, classification, and monitoring of dysfunction.[63] Table 11 gives a summary of this classification.

Meibomian gland dysfunction appears to increase the rate of deposit formation on hydrogel lenses.[64] The composition of the lens deposits is similar to that of the meibomian secretion.[65]

Rosacea is a common cause of blepharitis and meibomianitis. Rosacea can occur in patients of all ages but is most common in the 30- to 50-year-old group. This skin disease exhibits chronic papular and pustular dermatitis with erythema and hypertrophy of the sebaceous glands. It occurs most commonly on the nose, the forehead above the nose, and on the cheeks. Small telangiectatic spots are seen in these areas. The disease should be treated systemically with tetracycline.

Tear Film Consistency and Debris

Patients with decreased tear volume generally have more debris, probably mucous particles, floating in the tears. The tears will appear thicker and have a "gel" appearance. They will appear to move as a unit with lid movements.

Tear Meniscus

The major volume of the tears on the eye at any one time is in the tear menisci (also called tear prism or marginal tear strip) visible along the lid margins, which are especially visible when fluorescein is instilled (Plate 9). A careful examination of the tear menisci (usually the lower meniscus is evaluated) can be very enlightening. In patients

Table 11. Grades of Meibomian Gland Dysfunction

Grade	Orifices	Expression	Tear Film	Conjunctiva	Gland Appearance	Symptoms
0	Small holes	Clear fluid	No foaming Normal meniscus	No injection	Straight and uniform May not be visible	No symptoms
1	Orifices obvious Some pouting	May be abundance of clear fluid	May be some foaming	Trace injection Mild papillary hypertrophy Mild rose bengal stain	Some engorged	May have mild foreign body sensation Transient burning and dryness
2	Most obvious Some pouting and plugs	Abundance of fluid May be whitish yellow	Some foaming	Mild congestion and injection Increased papillary changes and rose bengal	Dilated and engorged Irregular shaped Discrete collections of lipid 1 or 2 microchalazia	Slight tearing, foreign body, burning, itching May report redness and crusting of lids
3	Increased pouting and plugs Inspissation of most	Expression difficult Often preceded by plug Whitish-yellow material	Foam centrally and at canthi Tear film debris Rapid BUT	Moderate congestion and irritation Moderate papillary hypertrophy Increased rose bengal	May be gross enlargement Multiple collections of lipid 3 or more microcha-lazia in lower lid	Moderate irritation, foreign body, tearing, mattering, redness, burning, itching Increased dryness
4	Increased pouting, plugging and compaction	Difficult Whitish-yellow, may be thick	Obvious foamy discharge Excessive debris Rapid BUT	Moderate to severe congestion and injection	Numerous collections of lipid Increased microchalazia	As in grade 3 Often history of recurrent chalazia

Source: Data from PJ Caroline, RT Kame. Meibomian Gland Dysfunction. In JA Silbert (ed), Anterior Segment Complications of Contact Lens Wear. New York: Churchill Livingstone, 1994.

with marginal dry eyes, this tear meniscus will be smaller than normal and often the edges of the meniscus will take on a scalloped appearance (Plate 10). In eyes with less tear production there may be almost no tear meniscus, particularly toward the canthi. The normal meniscus is about 0.3–0.6 mm in height.

By comparing the movement of debris deep in the tear meniscus to the movement of particles on the surface of the tear meniscus after a blink, the tear film viscosity can be estimated. With a very viscous tear film seen with drier eyes, the surface particles will move much faster than those in the meniscus.

Tear Film Break-Up Time

The tear film BUT is a valuable test of the integrity of the tear film. When the tear film thins, the aqueous layer is lost and the thickness reaches a point where the surface lipid layer touches the mucin layer. Likewise, if the mucin layer is deficient, the surface of the cornea is not wettable because of the lipid nature of the epithelial cells, and the tear film will break up very rapidly.

There are a couple of ways of measuring the BUT. One method is to instill fluorescein and then measure the time from a blink until the first dark spot (Plate 11) forms in the tear film. This is often called the invasive BUT. The other method is to reflect a pattern (such as a grid or line pattern) off the corneal surface and watch for the first distortion of the pattern. In this case no stain is used. This is often called the noninvasive BUT (NIBUT), since nothing is added to the tear film.

The technique used to measure the BUT is critical. When using the invasive BUT technique, it is important to minimize the disturbance of the tear film when instilling the fluorescein. The most accurate and repeatable results are obtained using a small drop (1–10 μl) of liquid fluorescein. The concentration of fluorescein recommended varies. Some recommend concentrations of 0.125%,[66] whereas others use a concentration as high as 5%.[67] In the average clinical practice it is common to use fluorescein strips. When fluorescein strips are used, they should be moistened with a buffered, nonpreserved saline, the excess solution shaken off, and the strip gently touched to the superior bulbar conjunctiva, inferior bulbar conjunctiva, or the lid margin with care being taken not to instill too much solution or cause excessive reflex tearing. After the fluorescein is instilled the patient should be instructed to blink normally two or three times. The patient is then told to stare straight ahead and not blink. The patient is told to keep the eyes open naturally and not to exaggerate the opening. The tear film is viewed with moderate magnification (10–20×) and a relatively wide parallelepiped (approximately 3 mm) using the cobalt filter over the light source and the yellow filter over the objective. The cornea is scanned from side to side. Using a stopwatch, the time from the blink until the first dark spot or streak is seen in the normal light green of the tear film is recorded as the BUT.

The lids should not be physically held open when measuring the BUT, as this will artificially decrease the BUT. Lemp and Hamill[68] found that holding the lids decreased the BUT an average of approximately 7 seconds. They also found that instilling proparacaine before the test decreased the BUT approximately 12 seconds. Any epithelial defect will result in a short BUT over that area and should not be taken as a deficiency of the tear film. A raised area or epithelial defect will cause "negative" staining—a small dark spot in the otherwise green fluorescein staining of the tear film. Repeated measurements of the BUT at one sitting will result in short BUTs. Likewise, if the BUT is measured a short time after a contact lens is removed, the BUT will be much shorter than normal because the contact lens will have prevented the normal spreading of the mucin layer over the corneal epithelium.

For normal persons the BUT is greater than 10 seconds. Rengstorff found approximately one-half of patients fell in the range of 10–30 seconds with 15% having BUTs of over 60 seconds and no normal person having a value below 10 seconds (Figure 18).[69] The first spot of break up was most commonly found in the temporal and inferior periphery

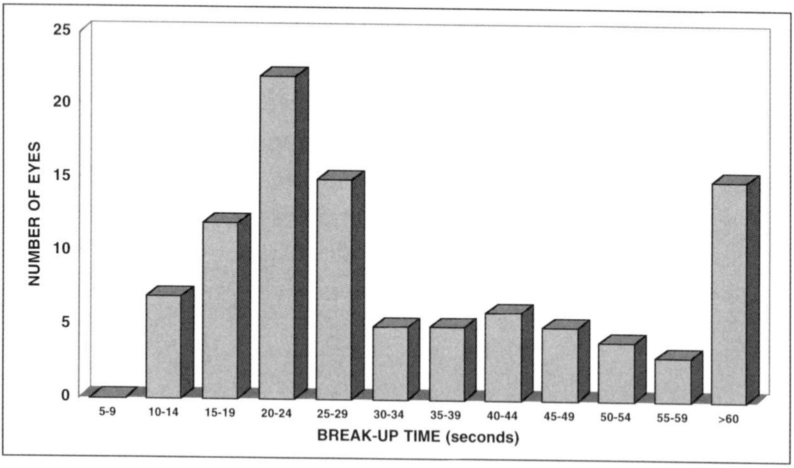

FIGURE 18. The distribution of tear film break-up times for a normal population of young adults. (Redrawn with permission from RH Rengstorff. The precorneal tear film: breakup time and location in normal subjects. Am J Optom Physiol Opt 1974;51:765.)

of the cornea. About two-thirds of the time the break up was in the periphery of the cornea as opposed to the central region. About two-thirds of the break-up areas were spots, with the remainder being streaks. There is usually little difference in the BUT between the two eyes; however, when measured on different days the variation was found to be considerable with a mean standard deviation of about 20 seconds.[70]

Marquardt et al. studied the difference in the BUT between using fluorescein strips and a 1-μl drop of fluorescein solution.[67] They found a marked increase in the BUT with the solution versus the strips (Figure 19).

It is generally accepted that invasive BUTs of less than 10 seconds should be considered abnormal and may indicate that a patient is not a good candidate for contact lens wear. However, many patients with 8- to 10-second BUTs do well.

The wearing of hydrogel lenses will cause the BUT on the corneal surface to be decreased for some time after lens removal. A decrease in BUT between that before fitting versus that measured within 10 minutes

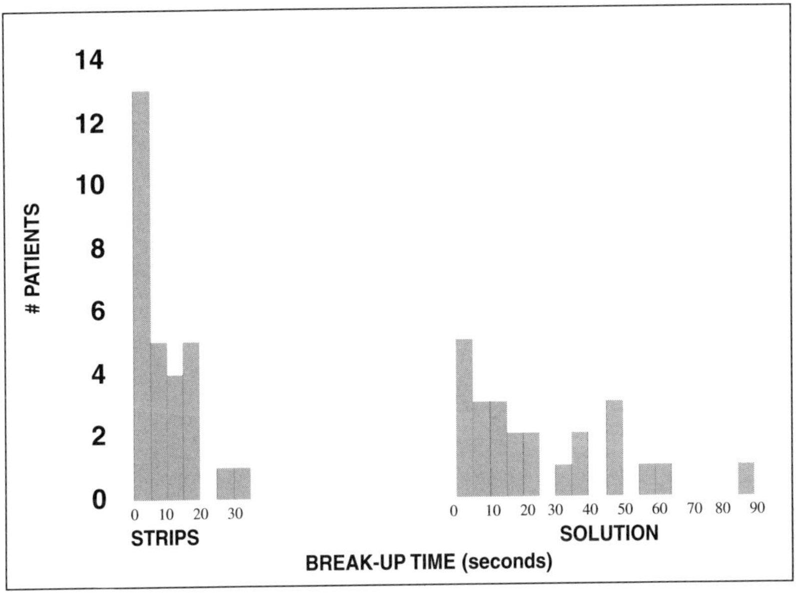

FIGURE 19. Comparison of the tear film break-up time (BUT) when fluorescein strips are used to the break-up time with a drop of fluorescein solution. The use of strips disrupts the tear film, shortening the time. (Modified from R Marquardt, R Stodtmeister, T Christ. Modification of Tear Film Break-up Time Test for Increased Reliability. In FJ Holly [ed], The Preocular Tear Film in Health, Disease, and Contact Lens Wear. Lubbock, TX: Dry Eye Institute, 1986;57.)

of hydrogel lens removal of 54% has been reported.[71] Faber et al. found that the recovery of the BUT (using the NIBUT technique) was significantly different than the nonwearing NIBUT for 15 minutes after lens removal and there was 95% of complete recovery in 25.8 minutes.[72]

The NIBUT is a more accurate measure of the true BUT since the tear film is not disturbed by the introduction of solution. Commonly a xeroscope or toposcope, an instrument consisting of a bowl with rings that is reflected from the corneal surface, is used.[73] The time from a blink until the first distortion of an area of the rings is used as the NIBUT. The normal NIBUT is about 40–60 seconds,[74] which is longer than the BUT measured using fluorescein (mean about 20 seconds). NIBUT values less than 20 seconds should be considered abnormal and an indication of a possible dry eye.

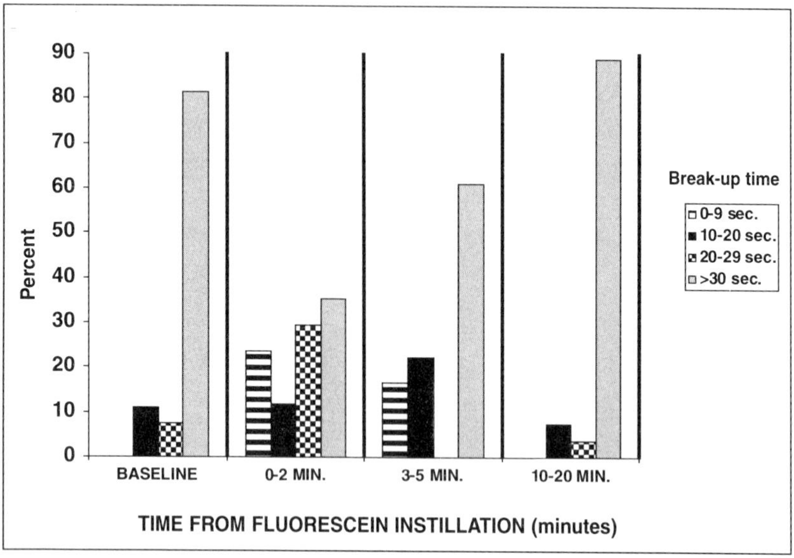

FIGURE 20. Duration of the effect of instilling fluorescein on the noninvasive break-up time (NIBUT). (Modified from LS Mengher, AJ Bron, SR Tonge, DJ Gilbert. A non-invasive instrument for clinical assessment of the pre-corneal tear film stability. Curr Eye Res 1985;4:1.)

A method of determining the NIBUT in the clinical setting is to measure what has been termed the tear thinning time (TTT). This is done by observing the keratometer mires and noting the time from a blink until the mires first become distorted.[75]

Figure 20 shows the BUT measured using the NIBUT technique before the instillation of fluorescein and then at different times after the fluorescein instillation.[73] As can be seen, the instillation of fluorescein shortened the BUT significantly. By 10–20 minutes after the instillation of the fluorescein the NIBUT was back to normal.

The BUT measurement is easily influenced by many factors that often result in variable values for the same patient. For this reason, the BUT found by one examiner may vary from that taken by a different individual. Therefore, care must be exercised and the same procedure used each time the measurement is made. If this is done, you will learn to know with your technique what is an abnormally low finding.

Summary of Break-Up Time Measurement

1. Measure break-up time before manipulating the lids or otherwise disturbing the tear film.
2. Instill a small amount of fluorescein. If using strips moistened with saline, shake off excess and lightly touch to eye to minimize irritation.
3. Have patient blink three or four times.
4. Have patient "stare" straight ahead and not blink (do not hold lids).
5. Time with a stopwatch from last blink to first break-up.
6. Use cobalt filter over light source and yellow filter over the objective.
7. Use a 3- to 4-mm–wide parallelepiped with minimum brightness to minimize tearing.
8. Scan cornea looking for break-up
9. If patient wears contact lenses, wait at least 15 minutes after lens removal.
10. Break-up time of greater than 10 seconds is usually satisfactory.

Fluorescein Staining

Looking for corneal staining with fluorescein before fitting a patient with contact lenses is important in detecting patients with dry-eye problems. Most marginal dry-eye patients will not have corneal staining; however, more moderate dry-eye patients will often show mild stipple staining of the cornea within the palpebral aperture (Plate 12). Obviously the more severe the dry eye, the greater the amount of staining.

Sometimes a fine line of corneal staining will be seen just within the palpebral aperture below the upper lid or above the lower lid. This may be caused by a blepharitis or meibomianitis but is often a finer line of staining than seen with these conditions. This fine line of staining may be caused by local drying along the corneal edge of the tear meniscus. The aqueous component of the tears in the meniscus will draw water from the tear film next to it by capillary attraction. This causes the normally occurring "black line" seen under high magnification along the tear meniscus when there is fluorescein in the tears. In patients with tear film problems this thinning may be enough to cause the corneal staining.

In marginal cases corneal staining is not seen with the first instillation of fluorescein. However, if fluorescein is instilled every 5 minutes for four or five times, rather dramatic staining can occur.[76] With one instillation of fluorescein 19% of the patients showed staining; after four instillations (15 minutes) 40% showed staining. They found that only 4% of patients who could successfully wear contact lenses showed significant staining, whereas 34% of patients who were previously unsuccessful in wearing contact lenses showed significant staining. Therefore, if drying is suspected, repeated instillations may demonstrate the problem. Caffery suggests instilling fluorescein in 2-minute intervals for 10 minutes.[77]

Fluorescein can be obtained either as a 1% or 2% solution or on a paper strip. Because of the potential for contamination of solutions and resultant infections, the strips are most commonly used, although the concentration can be better controlled with the solution. It is important to properly instill the fluorescein. The strip should be moistened with a buffered saline, the excess fluorescein and solution shaken off the strip, and the flat side of the strip touched against either the inferior or superior bulbar conjunctiva with minimal irritation of the eye. The strip should not be rubbed against the eye. Any irritation of the eye will cause reflex tearing and increase the chance of gathering incorrect information. Because of the problem of ocular irritation and disturbance of the tear film, some practitioners feel it is important to use the fluorescein solution for diagnosing dry eye problems. The appearance of the staining can be enhanced by using the cobalt filter in the biomicroscope (or a Wratten No. 47A or 47B filter) over the light source and a yellow filter (blue free) over the objective of the microscope (No. 12 or 15 Wratten filter or a similar yellow filter).

Rose Bengal Staining

Rose bengal staining is considered by many to be "the" diagnostic test for dry eye. This stain is a derivative of fluorescein that stains dead or degenerative cells and mucous strands but has been thought to not stain living epithelial cells.[78, 79] Feenstra and Tseng have found that rose bengal will stain living epithelial cells but that it is the tear film components such as albumin and mucin that prevent it from staining the cells.[80] Therefore, if the tear film is fully intact, there should be no staining with rose bengal, but with defects in the tear film rose bengal can reach the cell membranes and cause staining. Regardless of the mechanism, rose bengal is a very useful dye in detecting moderate and severe dry eyes.

Rose bengal is supplied both as a 1% solution and as a strip. The solution provides a more consistent concentration but the strips are convenient and can give satisfactory results. For those who use rose bengal only occasionally, the strips alleviate the concerns of contamination and outdated solutions.

Rose bengal causes considerably more stinging and discomfort on instillation than does fluorescein. The more extensive the staining, the greater the discomfort. Very little rose bengal is required to obtain sufficient staining. Therefore, only a minimal amount needs to be instilled. This can be done by teasing out a small wick of cotton on a cotton-tipped applicator, touching this to the stain and then touching the cotton wisp to the superior bulbar conjunctiva or tear meniscus. Likewise, the wooden end of the applicator can be dipped in solution or touched to the moistened strip to get a small amount of stain on it and then touched to the bulbar conjunctiva. If the strip is used to instill the stain directly, it should be moistened, the excess stain shaken off, and then the strip just barely touched to the inferior palpebral conjunctiva. Touching the strip to the inferior bulbar conjunctiva will cause staining in the touch area and mask any staining due to dryness. If a drop of stain is instilled, only a small drop (5 μl) should be used, and it should be placed on the superior bulbar conjunctiva as the patient looks down. The patient should be instructed to blink several times after the instillation and about a minute should pass before the amount of staining is evaluated. The staining will be more visible under red-free light (use a green filter). Caution should be used to prevent getting rose bengal on the patient's clothing, as it can cause permanent stains.

Since rose bengal stains dead or degenerating cells or epithelial cells not protected by mucin, the pattern of staining in patients with dry eyes will be in the area of the eye normally exposed and not those areas under the lids. Both the cornea and conjunctiva take up the red stain with a fine stipple pattern observed (Plate 13). Any strands of mucous present will also stain.

Staining can be graded on a 0–3 scale (0, no staining; 1, mild; 2, moderate; and 3, severe) for the nasal conjunctiva, cornea, and temporal conjunctiva. For example, the staining might be graded nasal conjunctiva, 1; cornea, 1; and temporal conjunctiva, 2.

Because rose bengal and fluorescein stain different anomalies, both stains should be used when examining a patient suspected of having a tear film problem. Both stains can be instilled at the same time.

Other Vital Stains

A number of different stains have been used to highlight corneal and conjunctival defects as well as mucus.

Fluorexon

Fluorexon is a high-molecular-weight fluorescein developed for use with hydrogel contact lenses because it is only very slowly absorbed by these lenses. It is not a good stain for showing corneal or conjunctival defects because it is not readily absorbed by the defects.

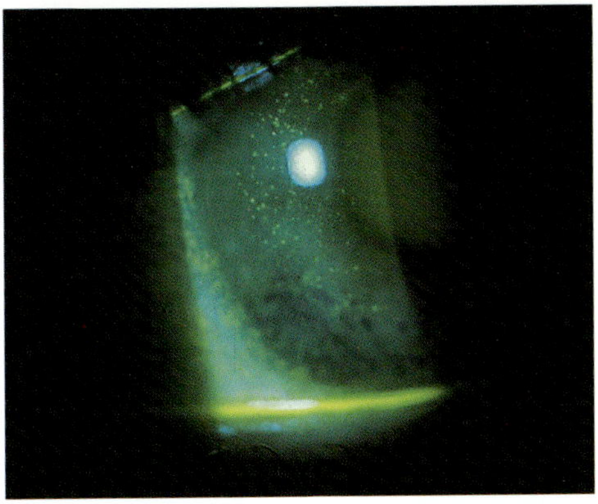

PLATE 1. Photograph of corneal staining resulting from dehydration through a high water content lens. Fluorescein has been instilled.

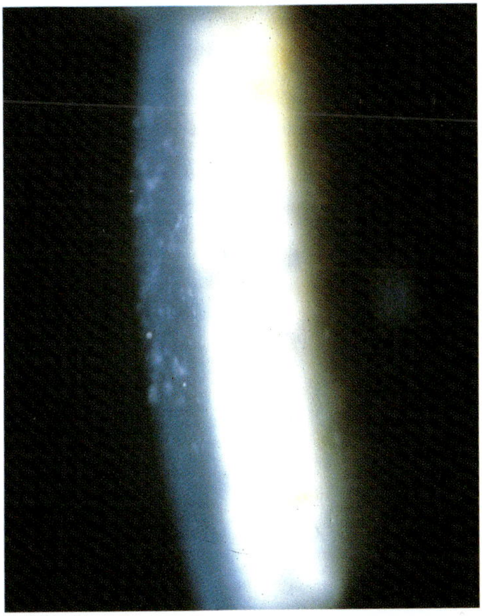

PLATE 2. Photograph of corneal epithelial disruption from dehydration through a high water content hydrogel lens. No stain was instilled.

PLATE 3. Inferior, mid-peripheral arcuate staining from desiccation with the wearing of a hydrogel lens.

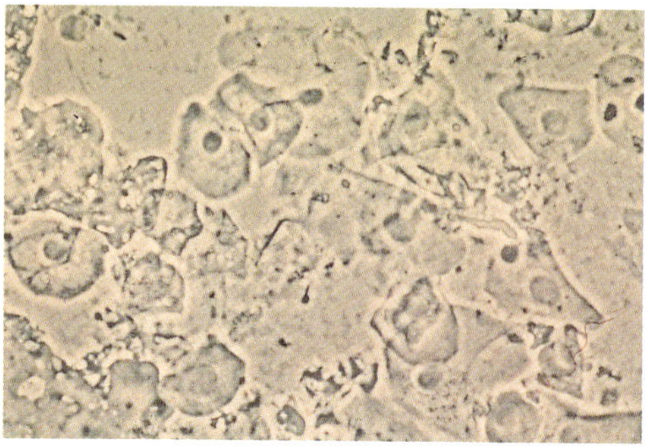

PLATE 4. Cells and debris on the back surface of an extended-wear hydrogel lens.

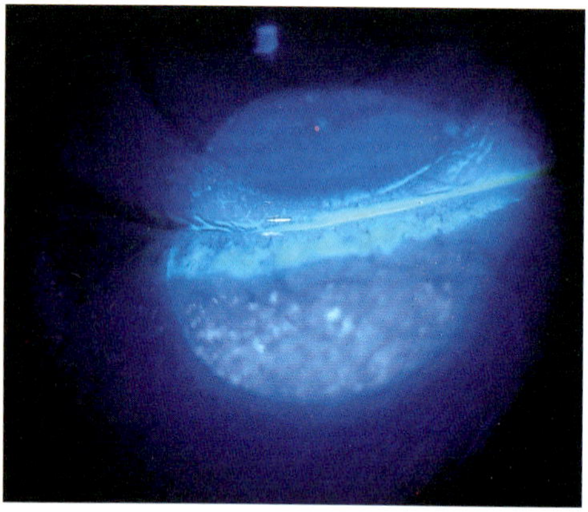

PLATE 5. Dried mucoid material along the lower lid margin. This is a typical finding in patients with dry eye.

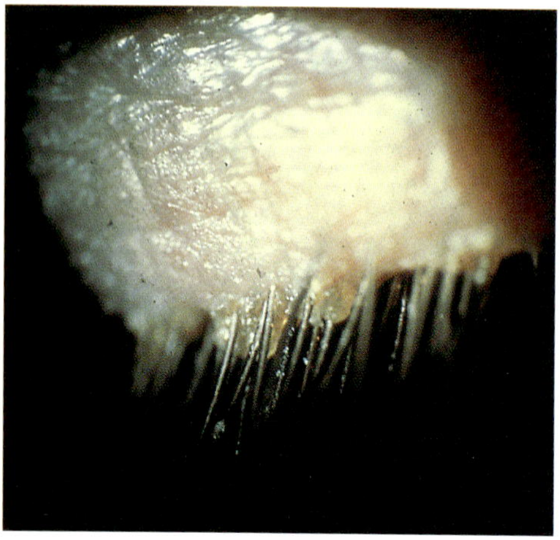

PLATE 6. Collarettes on the lashes of a patient with blepharitis. (Courtesy of Dr. Victor Malinovsky.)

PLATE 7. Inferior keratitis as the result of blepharitis. (Courtesy of Dr. Victor Malinovsky.)

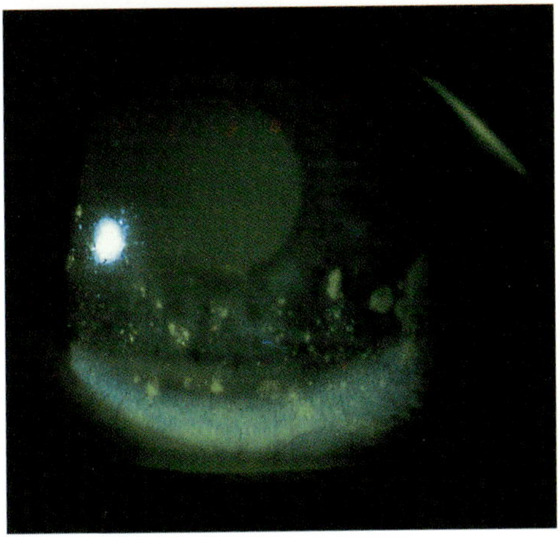

PLATE 8. Pouting at the opening of the meibomian glands.

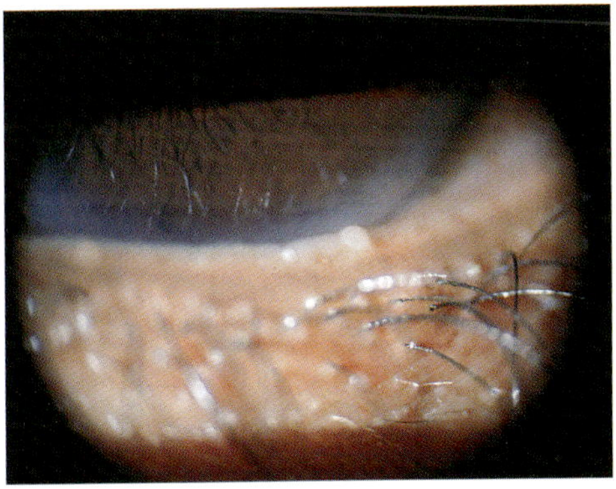

PLATE 9. A normal tear meniscus along the lower lid margin.

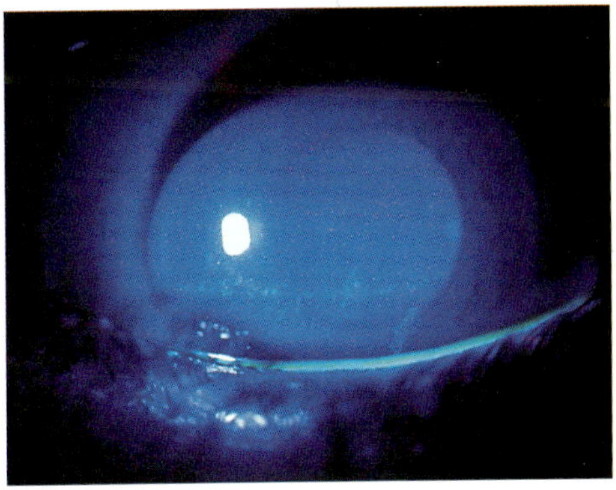

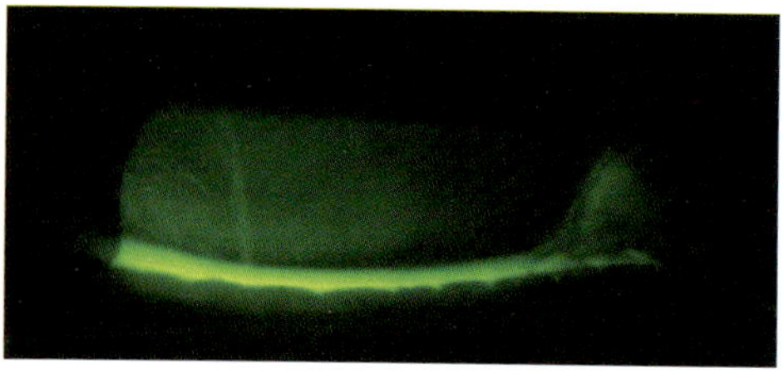

PLATE 10. The tear meniscus of a patient with a marginal dry eye showing scalloping along the edge of the meniscus.

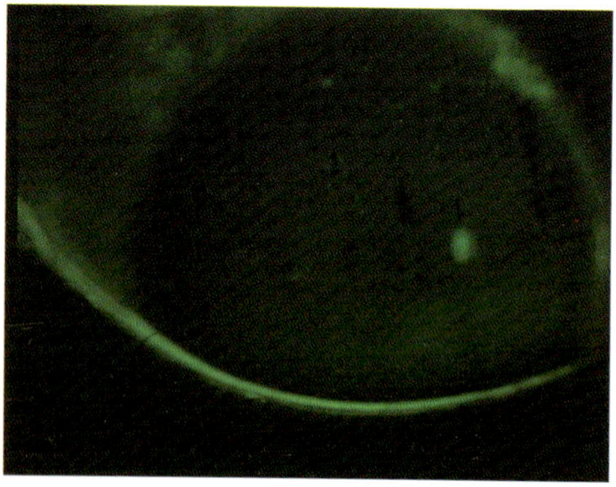

PLATE 11. Dark spots indicating break-up of the tear film.

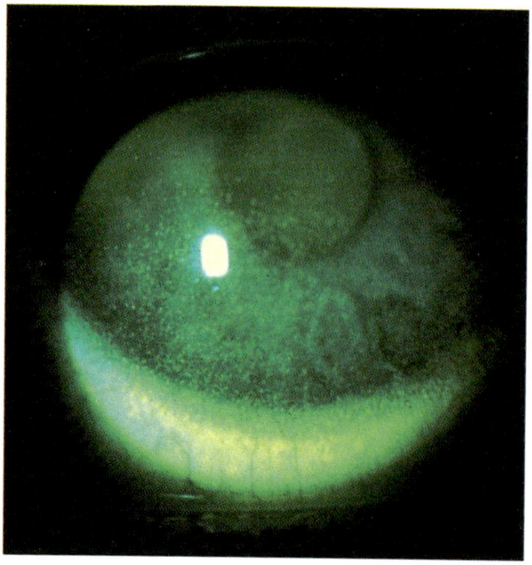

PLATE 12. Typical corneal staining on the inferior cornea of a patient with a moderately dry eye.

PLATE 13. Rose bengal staining on a patient with a moderately dry eye. (Courtesy of Dr. Victor Malinovsky.)

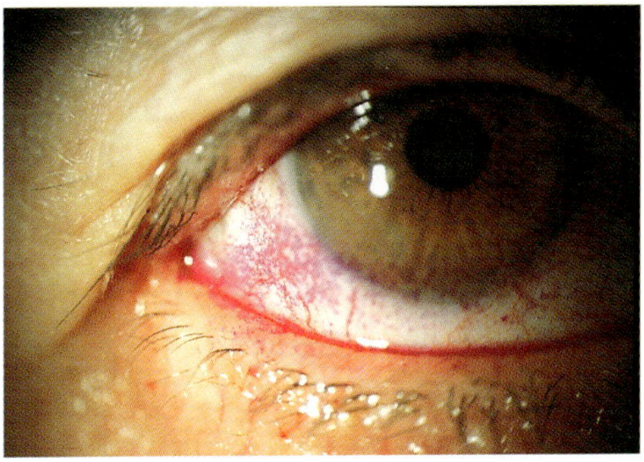

PLATE 14. Technique of using a cotton-tipped applicator and digital pressure to force material from the meibomian glands.

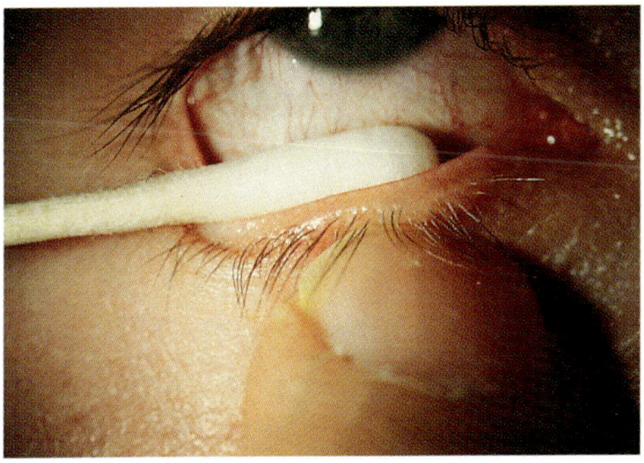

PLATE 15. A collagen implant held in tweezers ready to be inserted into the punctum.

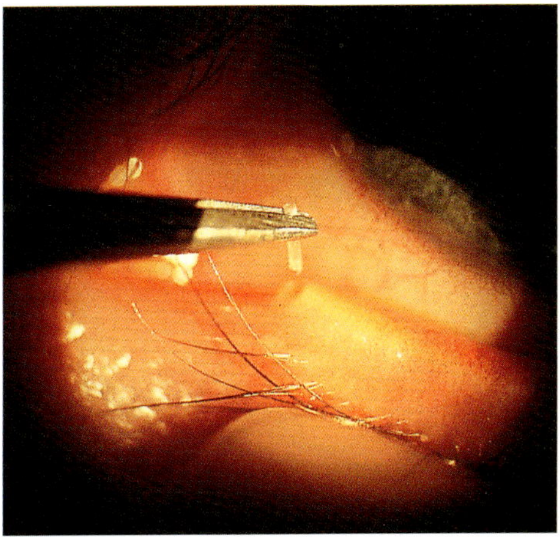

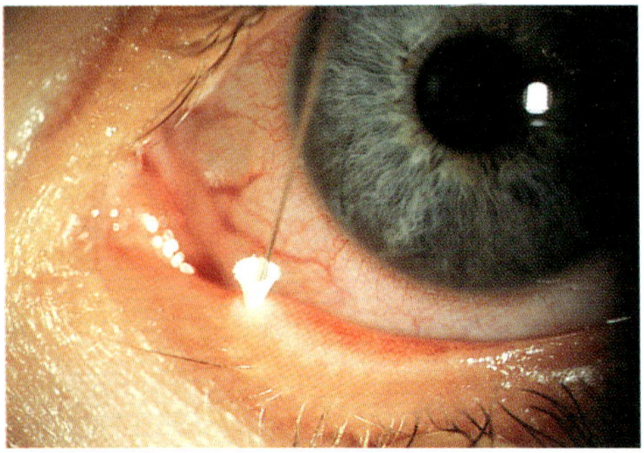

PLATE 16. The first step in inserting a Herrick lacrimal plug—insertion into the punctum.

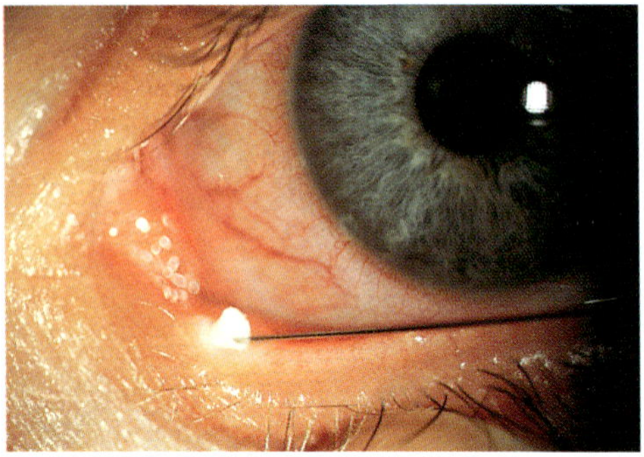

PLATE 17. The holder of the lacrimal plug is turned parallel to the lid margin to push the plug into the canaliculus.

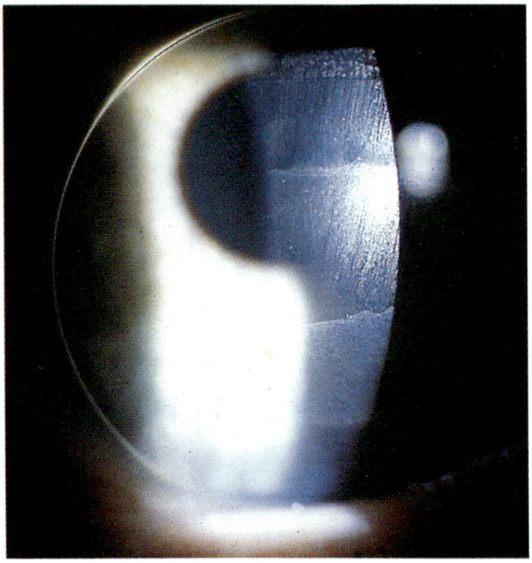

PLATE 18. The dry surface of a rigid gas-permeable lens that can occur between blinks.

PLATE 19. The build-up of a coating on the inside surface of a rigid gas-permeable lens as seen under magnification. (Courtesy of Dr. Christopher Snyder.)

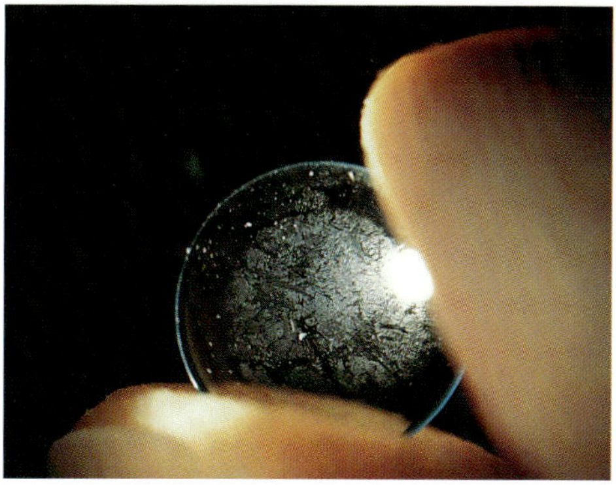

PLATE 20. The corneal staining that occurs with the use of a lens with significant build-up on the inside surface.

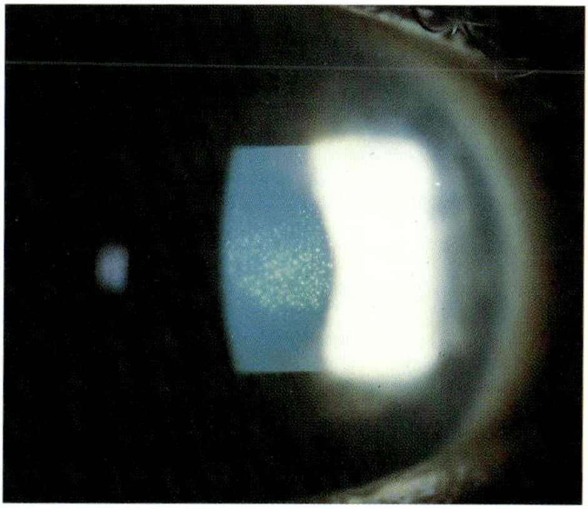

PLATE 21. A. Grade 1 peripheral corneal staining showing a few spots of stippling.

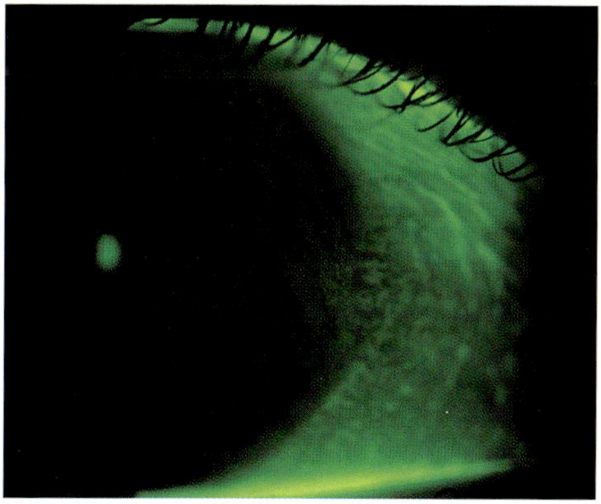

A

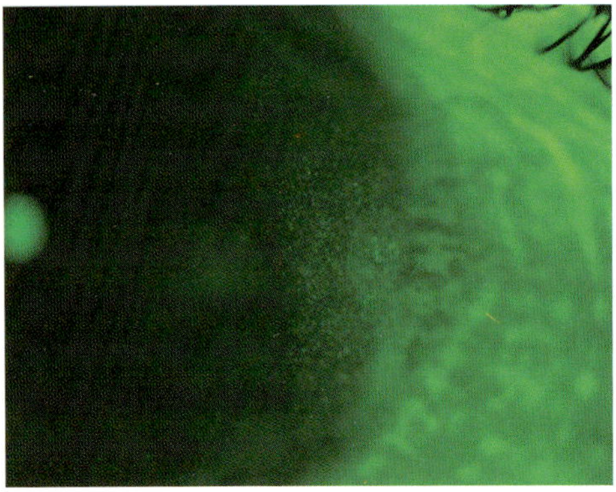

B

PLATE 21. (continued). B. Grade 2 peripheral staining.

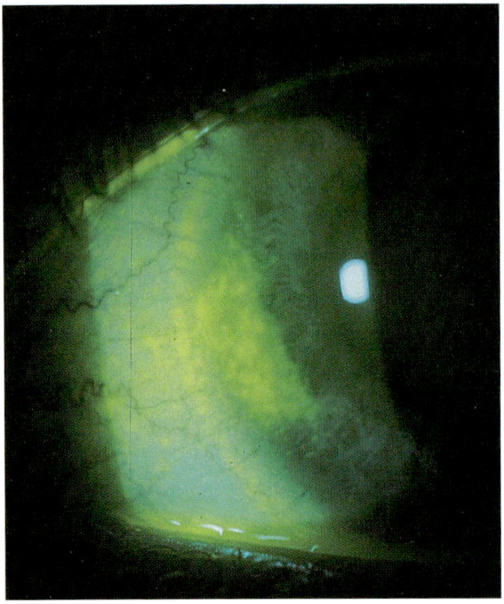

C

C. Grade 3 staining showing coalesced staining.

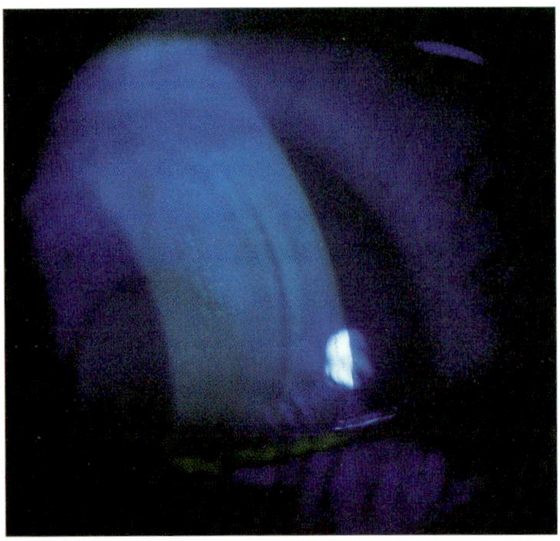

PLATE 22. An impression ring left on the cornea from an adherent extended-wear rigid gas-permeable lens.

Lissamine Green

Lissamine green is a stain that has been used to stain the cornea and conjunctiva.[81] It has been used in foods. Used as a 1% solution, it stains the cornea and conjunctiva very similarly to a 1% solution of rose bengal.[82] The staining is easier to see against the conjunctival blood vessels and does not sting on instillation as does rose bengal.

Alcian Blue

Used in a 1% solution, alcian blue stains mucus, and with normal eyes a few fine spots of blue staining will be seen on the cornea and conjunctiva. With dry eyes the staining is more pronounced and is similar to that seen with rose bengal staining except alcian blue only stains mucus. Alcian blue should not be used on eyes with full-thickness epithelial abrasions or defects because it might permanently stain the stroma.

Schirmer Test

The Schirmer test uses a filter paper strip 5 mm wide by 35 mm long to absorb tears. One end is bent over and placed under the temporal portion of the lower lid and left in place for 5 minutes. With no anesthetic (Schirmer I test), over 10 mm of the strip should be moistened in 5 minutes. With the use of an anesthetic (Schirmer II or Jones test), over 5 mm of the strip should be moistened by the tears in 5 minutes. When using an anesthetic, the examiner should wait at least 2–3 minutes after instilling the anesthetic before doing the test to allow excess solution to escape. Blotting excess solution from the canthi should be done before the test if excess solution is present. Some practitioners use shorter times, for example 2.5 minutes and double the length of wetting. This can give erroneous findings, since there is more wetting the first minute or two than later because of the reservoir of tears in the tear meniscus that is initially absorbed.

The general theory has been that there was a basal level of tear production that was independent of stimulation (the Schirmer II test would measure this). However, it is now thought that all tearing is the result of stimulation. The evidence for this is the lack of tear production under general anesthesia.

The Schirmer test is quite variable because of the irritation to the eye when doing the test. It is not a very good test for a marginal dry eye that creates the problems with normal contact lens wear.

Impression Cytology

Impression cytology is a technique in which a piece of cellulose acetate filter paper is pressed against the conjunctiva, which removes the surface layer of cells. By examining this layer of cells under the microscope the health of the conjunctival surface can be evaluated.

Slightly varying techniques have been used to collect the cells. Nelson uses 0.25-inch diameter circular filter paper, which he applies to the bulbar conjunctiva with 40–45 g of pressure using an ophthalmodynamometer.[83] He collects specimens from the temporal, nasal, and superior bulbar conjunctiva. He also collects a sample from the inferior palpebral conjunctiva using 70–75 g pressure on the filter paper. Samples can also be obtained in a simpler manner by just pressing the filter paper against the conjunctiva with a glass rod[84] or similar device, although this does not give consistent results. Connors has found that taking three consecutive samples from the same spot on the conjunctiva will result in a better specimen on the third sample, since the first two samples remove the tear film, mucin layer, and so forth, allowing the third sample to collect more cells.[85] The filter paper pieces are placed on a microscope slide and fixed with a spray fixative and stained with hematoxylin and periodic acid–Schiff (PAS) stains. The specimens are then dried and examined.

Both regular surface epithelial cells and goblet cells will be seen on the samples with the epithelial cells staining blue and the mucin in the goblet cells staining red. The size and condition of the epithelial cells is important. Normal epithelial cells are small and round.

Table 12. Grading Scale for Impression Cytology

Grade	*Goblet Cells (count per mm)*	*Nuclei/Cytoplasm Ratio*	*Appearance of Epithelial Cells*
0	>500	1:2	Small, round with esophilic staining cytoplasm; large, basophilic staining nuclei
1	350–500	1:3	Slightly larger and more polygonal epithelium; nuclei slightly smaller
2	100–350	1:4 to 1:5	Epithelial cells larger and more polygonal; occasional multinucleated cells
3	<100	>1:6	Epithelial cells large and polygonal; basophilic staining cytoplasm

Source: Data from JD Nelson. Impression cytology. Cornea 1988;7:71.

With dryness they become larger, whereas the nuclei become smaller. With dry-eye problems the number of goblet cells decreases. Nelson recommended the grading scale in Table 12 for conjunctival impression cytology.

Any finding of grade 2 or greater is considered abnormal. The findings with respect to the number of cells will vary with technique.

Basic Objective Examination for Marginal Dry Eye

1. Examine lids for blepharitis.
2. Examine lids for meibomian gland dysfunction.
3. Evaluate the tear meniscus and tear film.
4. Measure the break-up time.
5. Determine if there is any fluorescein or rose bengal staining.

Other Useful Tear Film Tests

There are many tests that have been used experimentally or in special circumstances to study the tear film or diagnose tear film–related problems. Because of the lack of normal clinical applicability, these are not covered in this text. However, there are a number of tests that are more commonly used in specialized practices of which the eye care clinician should be aware even though they may not be performed in the primary care practice. Following is a short description of these tests.

Phenol Red Thread Test

The phenol red thread test consists of using a two-ply cotton thread 70 mm in length that has been soaked in phenol red dye. Phenol red is a pH-sensitive dye that stains the thread yellow but turns red when tears are absorbed. Three millimeters of the end of the thread is bent over and placed under the temporal portion of the lower lid as is done with a Schirmer strip. The patient is then asked to close his or her eyes. The thread is left in place 15 seconds. When removed the length of the thread from the crimped position that has turned red is measured. A mean average wetting length of 16.7 mm (from a study of 1,890 patients) was found for normal patients, with wetting lengths less than 9 mm considered abnormal. Fifty-eight percent of patients with wetting lengths of less than 9 mm had dryness symptoms.[86] The advantages of this test are that it is less irritating to the patient and takes less time. Because of the short time period used, it may actually be primarily measuring the tear volume on the eye at the time of the test and not the secretion rate.

Osmolarity

The osmotic pressure of the tear film will increase because of evaporation of water, leaving a higher concentration of ions in the tear film. Thus, if there is a reduced production of tears with the same evaporation rate, the osmotic pressure will increase. This is measured by taking a small sample of tears (0.2 μl) and using a nanoliter osmometer.[87] Normal patients have average values of 302 ± 6.3 mOsm/liter, with 312 mOsm/liter or greater considered to be abnormal and an indication of decreased tear production.[88] This is a very sensitive test and is felt to be better than most of the clinical tests presently used. However, it does require specialized equipment and is a relatively difficult technique to perform.

Fluorescein Dilution Test

The rate at which a dye is lost from the inferior tear meniscus has been used as an indicator of the rate of tear production and flow. Norn uses a mixture of 1% rose bengal and 1% fluorescein.[82] He places a small drop (10 µl) of the dye solution onto the eye. Then the patient is told to keep the eyes open and just blink normally but not to squeeze the lids. After 5 minutes the color of the meniscus is compared with known dilutions of the dye solution in capillary tubes (dilutions of 1:4, red; 1:16, pale red; 1:64, orange; 1:256, pale orange; 1:1,024, yellow; 1:4,096, pale yellow). For normal subjects the color of the tear meniscus becomes yellow. For dry-eye patients the meniscus remains red or bright orange.

Fluorophotometry can also be used to measure the rate of loss of fluorescein from the eye, but very specialized research equipment is required.[89]

Lacrimal Equilibration Time

The lacrimal equilibration time (LET) test consists of placing a drop of a viscous artificial tear solution in the lower cul-de-sac and measuring the time from the instillation until the visual acuity returns to the baseline value. Using a drop of Celluvisc (Allergan, Inc.), Lavaux and Keller found that patients with normal tear films required an average of 2.6 minutes for the visual acuity to return whereas patients with symptoms of dryness required 10.8 minutes for the acuity to return.[90] More testing is required to determine if this is a reliable clinical test.

Lactoferrin Immunoassay Testing

Lactoferrin is a protein in the tear film and is an important antibacterial component of the tears. It is secreted by the lacrimal gland and can be a good indicator of tear production. There is a commercial test (Lactoplate, Eagle Vision, Memphis, TN) used to determine the concentration in the tears. A small, round piece of filter paper is placed in the lower cul-de-sac to absorb the tears. It is then removed, blotted, and placed on agar gel, which contains the antibody. The gel is allowed to set for 72 hours and then the diameter of the precipitate ring is measured to determine the level of lactoferrin. Even though this is a repeatable test, it is relatively expensive and waiting 3 days for the results is a problem.

Lysozyme

Lysozyme is one of the major proteins in the tears and is an important antibacterial agent. It can also be measured using laboratory techniques similar to those used to measure lactoferrin. Because of the time and difficulty in measuring lysozyme, it is not a viable, routine clinical test.

Prediction

A modified McMonnies questionnaire and a series of objective tests were given to two groups of contact lens patients[57]: one group of 32 patients with the symptom of dryness with hydrogel lens wear and a second group of 26 patients without the symptom. In response to the question, "Do you regard your eyes as being unusually sensitive to cigarette smoke, smog, air conditioning, or central heating?" 56% of those with dryness symptoms indicated a problem, with only 12% of asymptomatic patients indicating the problem (Figure 21). Likewise, on the question, "Do you experience dryness of the nose, mouth, throat, chest, or vagina?" 13% of those with contact lens dryness indicated "often" with none of the asymptomatic patients indicating

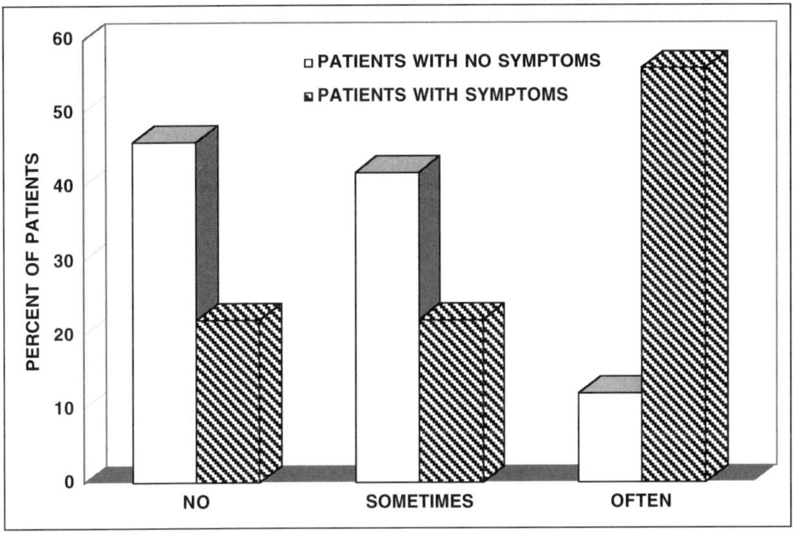

FIGURE 21. The responses of hydrogel contact lens patients with no symptoms (open bars) and those with dryness symptoms (shaded bars) to the question, "Do you regard your eyes as being unusually sensitive to cigarette smoke, smog, air conditioning, or central heating?" (Redrawn with permission from GE Lowther. Comparison of hydrogel contact lens patients with and without the symptoms of dryness. ICLC 1993;20:191.)

this problem occurred often (Figure 22). For the question about irritation on awakening, 21% of the patients with dryness symptoms indicated they often or always had this irritation (Figure 23). As one would expect, the majority (94%) of patients with contact lens dryness symptoms used rewetting drops. With the objective tests, there was a significant difference in the BUT with longer times for the asymptomatic group (12.7 ± 7.8 seconds versus 8.6 ± 6.7 seconds). There was also a difference in the Lactoplate results, with the asymptomatic group having higher levels (13.5 ± 2.67 mm) than the symptomatic patients (11.92 ± 2.69 mm). However, because of the small difference and the size of the standard deviation, it would be difficult to use this as a diagnostic tool. There was also a greater amount of staining with the symptomatic group, although many of these patients did not have staining.

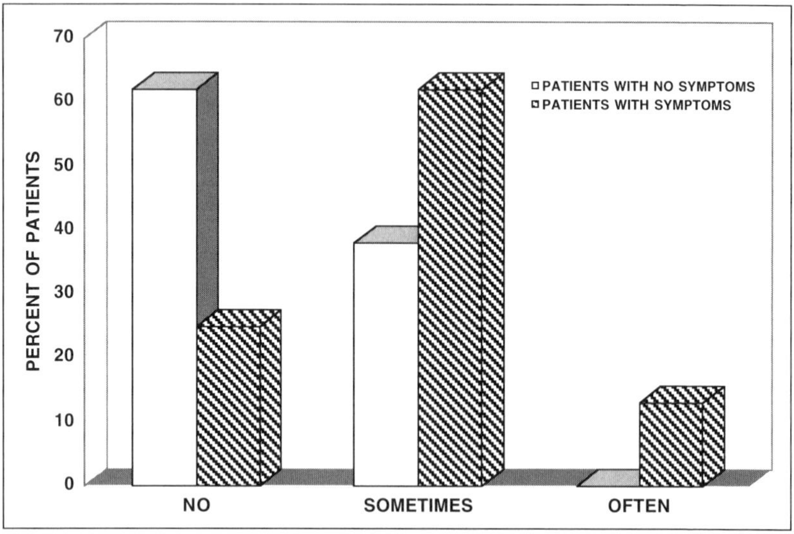

FIGURE 22. The responses of hydrogel contact lens patients with no symptoms (open bars) and those with dryness symptoms (shaded bars) to the question, "Do you experience dryness of the nose, mouth, throat, chest, or vagina?" (Redrawn from GE Lowther. Comparison of hydrogel contact lens patients with and without the symptoms of dryness. ICLC 1993;20:191.)

A study of 214 hydrogel lens wearers also found that the McMonnies's questionnaire was a good predictor of dryness symptoms with lens wear.[91]

From the above it can be seen that it is possible to predict at least some of the patients who may develop drying symptoms with hydrogel lens wear during the prefitting examination. Using the dry-eye questionnaire and doing a good prefitting examination looking at the lids, lashes, BUT, staining, tear prism, and debris in the tears is beneficial. No one test is definitive, but taken together often enough information can be garnered to make the prediction.

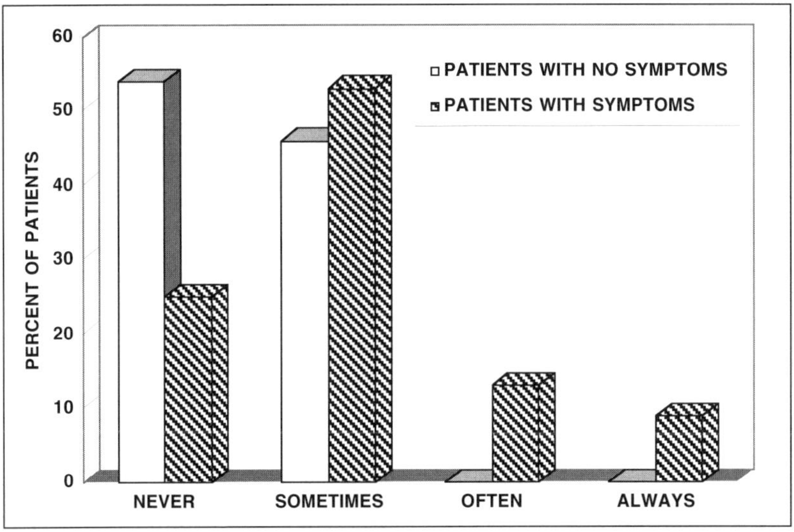

FIGURE 23. The responses of hydrogel contact lens patients with no symptoms (open bars) and those with dryness symptoms (shaded bars) to the question, "Do you have eye irritation as you wake from sleep?" (Redrawn from GE Lowther. Comparison of hydrogel contact lens patients with and without the symptoms of dryness. ICLC 1993;20:191.)

Handling Hydrogel Lens Patients with Contact Lens–Tear Film Problems

The situation the clinician must deal with each day is solving the patient's problem. What should we do with a patient with dryness symptoms or corneal staining from drying? When are signs and symptoms severe enough to merit lens changes? When should contact lens wear be discontinued?

Rewetting Drops

One of the most common recommendations given contact lens patients with drying symptoms is to use rewetting drops.[2] The problem with rewetting drops is that patients have relief from the symptoms for only 10–20 minutes after they are used and then the symptoms rapidly return. Golding et al. found that the effect of three different lubricants lasted less than 5 minutes.[92] The BUT on the lens surface was back to baseline values in less than 5 minutes. There were no differences between the three lubricants used.

Efron et al. studied the effect of instilling two different lubricants and saline drops on the water content of hydrogel lenses.[93] They found no difference in lens hydration levels among the three solutions, and the lens hydration levels were no better than before instillation of the drops (Figure 24). The lens hydration was measured 20 minutes after the last drop was instilled. In the same study the patients rated the comfort equally improved with all the drops (saline was as good as the lubricants). The reported increase in comfort could be a placebo effect, since the study was done in 6-hour time periods and the patient completed the comfort rating 10 minutes after the last drop.

Different tonicity solutions, hypotonic or hypertonic, have been used to attempt to rehydrate hydrogel lenses on the eye. A study by

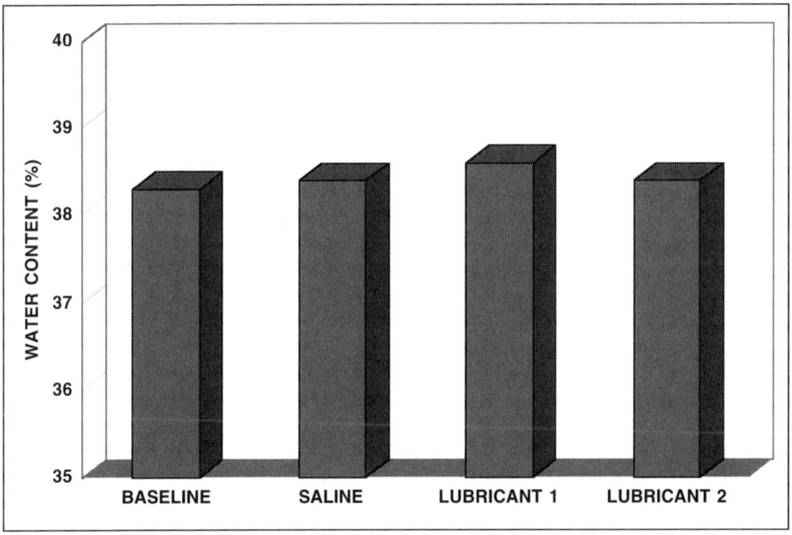

FIGURE 24. Effect of saline and two different lubricants on the hydration level of hydrogel lenses. No significant difference from the baseline value was found. (Modified with permission from N Efron, TR Golding. The effect of soft lens lubricants on symptoms and lens dehydration. CLAO J 1991;17:114.)

Aiello and Insler, however, found no difference in lens hydration when Hypotears (Ciba Vision), a 224 mOsm/liter solution, was used compared with Adsorbonac 2% (Alcon), a 670 mOsm/liter solution.[94] Normal saline is a 289 mOsm/liter solution.

There is not much difference between the effectiveness of the different commercial rewetting drops or lubricants; in fact, saline appears to be just as effective in many cases. There has been a concern that preservatives in rewetting drops may be detrimental with respect to the solution effectiveness and comfort. In studying some 10 different commercially available drops Caffery and Josephson found little difference between most of them.[95] The nonpreserved solutions ranked highest with respect to comfort. With a number of nonpreserved solutions on the market, it is easy to recommend their use.

In general, the effectiveness of the presently available rewetting and lubricating drops are short lived and not a very satisfactory solution to the patients' problems. It may be that the drops actually make the situation worse, since they may disrupt the oily layer of the tear film allowing for accelerated evaporation.

Lens Soaks

Rewetting drops do not rehydrate lenses because the solution is washed out of the eye so quickly. It is known that, because of the efficient drainage system, most pharmaceutical agents usually do not reside on the eye long enough to be adequately absorbed. A drop of solution is washed away in minutes. If a solution containing a preservative, such as benzalkonium chloride, is dropped onto an eye wearing a hydrogel lens, there is seldom any problem. On the other hand, if the same hydrogel lens is soaked in the solution, the concentration of the preservative in the lens can become quite high. When placed on the eye, a chemical keratitis will result.

Since rewetting solutions are quickly washed away, an alternative to using them would be to have the patient remove the lenses and soak them in saline or disinfectant solution to rehydrate them. If, for example, the initial symptoms take 3–5 hours to become a problem, the patient may be able to get another 3–5 hours of comfortable wear after a soak. My clinical impression is that many patients find a short 10–20 second soak of the lens in the palm of the hand sufficient to give a much longer comfort period than drops on the lens on the eye. A good clinical trial is required to determine how effective this is and under what circumstances it works the best.

Environment

Since it has been shown that lenses tend to dehydrate more in low humidity and windy conditions, patients with symptoms should be questioned about their environments. If they work near a heating duct, do not have a humidifier, or have other conditions that can be changed to improve their comfort, this is an easy and effective method of solving their problem. Patients who must work under such conditions may have to be fitted with other lens types to minimize the problem.

Patients should be warned that under certain conditions they may have problems. For example, if they live in a relatively humid climate they may develop some symptoms when they travel to dry areas. Fatt and Rocher looked at the effect of temperature and humidity conditions on lens wear.[96] They used the concept of the driving pressure of water leaving the eye to determine favorable and unfavorable temperature and humidity conditions for contact lens wear. The net driving pressure of water leaving the eye is the driving pressure of water leaving minus the driving pressure of water returning from the air. The returning pressure is called the water vapor pressure in air and is easily calculated from temperature and humidity. As a result of the substances in the tears and the matrix of a hydrogel lens that inhibits water flow, they estimated the net driving pressure to be 0.75 of pure water vapor pressure at eye temperature minus the water vapor pressure in air. The lower this calculated value, the less dehydration there would be. Low values would occur with higher humidities and temperatures. They chose 20 mm Hg of evaporation driving pressure or higher as conditions in which many patients would have dehydration problems. Based on this value they developed a table for different cities around the world indicating the months during which on average patients should be comfortable or uncomfortable. Table 13 lists a few of the cities indicating estimated comfort or discomfort from dehydration.

Individuals who regularly take long airline flights will often complain of dryness because of the low humidity. It might be recommended that they remove their lenses on such flights.

New Lenses

Since surface deposits may become hydrophobic, coated lenses will dry rapidly, causing increased symptoms of dryness and discomfort. Such lenses should be replaced. If a patient has signs and symptoms of a marginal dry eye, a condition that is known to increase the rate

Table 13. Driving Pressure for Evaporation of Water from Tears and Hydrogel Lenses (in mm Hg) in Various Cities by Month*

City	*Jan*	*Feb*	*Mar*	*Apr*	*May*	*Jun*	*Jul*	*Aug*	*Sep*	*Oct*	*Nov*	*Dec*
Albuquerque	24	24	23	23	22	21	18	16	22	23	23	23
	U	U	U	U	U	U	F	F	U	U	U	U
Boston	23	23	23	22	17	15	14	14	14	16	21	23
	U	U	U	U	F	F	F	F	F	F	U	U
Buenos Aires	11	11	11	14	17	16	16	16	16	16	15	12
	F	F	F	F	F	F	F	F	F	F	F	F
Calcutta	14	14	10	6	3	1	1	1	1	4	11	13
	F	F	F	F	F	F	F	F	F	F	F	F
Chicago	23	23	23	21	17	12	12	12	14	18	22	23
	U	U	U	U	F	F	F	F	F	F	U	U
Edmonton	25	25	24	22	20	18	16	16	19	21	24	24
	U	U	U	U	U	F	F	F	F	U	U	U
Jerusalem	20	29	19	19	19	18	16	15	16	17	18	19
	U	U	F	F	F	F	F	F	F	F	F	F
Las Vegas	24	23	24	24	24	23	20	20	23	23	23	24
	U	U	U	U	U	U	U	U	U	U	U	U
London	21	21	21	20	19	17	17	16	17	19	20	21
	U	U	U	U	F	F	F	F	F	F	U	U
Manila	7	7	8	6	5	2	2	3	3	4	5	5
	F	F	F	F	F	F	F	F	F	F	F	F
Miami	14	14	14	10	9	8	6	6	6	9	11	14
	F	F	F	F	F	F	F	F	F	F	F	F

Montreal	24	24	23	21	19	15	13	14	17	20	22	24
	U	U	U	U	F	F	F	F	F	U	U	U
New Orleans	17	18	16	14	12	10	8	8	8	13	16	18
	F	F	F	F	F	F	F	F	F	F	F	F
New York	23	23	22	20	18	14	12	11	14	16	21	23
	U	U	U	U	F	F	F	F	F	F	U	U
Paris	21	21	21	20	19	16	16	16	17	18	20	20
	U	U	U	U	F	F	F	F	F	F	U	U
Rio de Janeiro	6	6	6	8	10	11	12	12	11	11	9	8
	F	F	F	F	F	F	F	F	F	F	F	F
San Francisco	19	20	20	18	17	16	15	15	15	16	18	20
	F	U	U	F	F	F	F	F	F	F	F	U
Sydney	12	12	12	15	17	18	19	19	18	16	15	13
	F	F	F	F	F	F	F	F	F	F	F	F
Vancouver	21	21	20	19	18	16	14	15	16	18	20	20
	U	U	U	F	F	F	F	F	F	F	U	U
Washington DC	23	23	23	20	17	13	10	9	14	16	21	23
	U	U	U	U	F	F	F	F	F	F	U	U

*Values of 20 mm Hg and above are considered unfavorable (U) conditions and those less than 20 mm Hg are considered favorable (F).
Source: Data from I Fatt, P Rocher. Contact lens performance in different climates. Optometry Today (London), January 1994, pp 26–31.

of deposit formation, then putting the patient on a frequent replacement schedule is prudent.

Solutions

Some patients have symptoms of dryness that appear to be related to a sensitivity to preservatives in solutions rather than a true drying or dehydration of the lens. If this is suspected, the patient can change to a preservative-free care regimen and solutions. Some practitioners routinely change all patients with dryness symptoms to nonpreserved solutions. A well-defined study is required to determine the degree and magnitude of the problem caused by preservatives.

Treatment of Meibomian Gland Dysfunction and Blepharitis

The aggressiveness of the treatment of meibomianitis and blepharitis depends on the practitioner and the severity of the problem. In milder cases, putting the patient on lid hygiene at home is sufficient. The more aggressive approach to treating meibomianitis is for the practitioner to express the glands in the office on a regular schedule and to prescribe systemic medications in addition to having the patient carry out lid hygiene at home.

In-office meibomian gland expression for meibomian gland dysfunction has been described by Korb et al.[61, 97] Topical anesthetic is dropped into the cul-de-sac. The eyelid margins are scrubbed with a cotton-tipped applicator soaked in the anesthetic solution to remove debris and further anesthetize the lid margins. The patient is instructed to look up and the lower lid is pulled away from the globe. The cotton-tipped applicator is placed in the lower cul-de-sac against the lower tarsal conjunctiva adjacent to a meibomian gland near its orifice. Digital pressure is applied with the thumb to the skin of the lid while the cotton-tipped applicator is held behind the lid to compress the gland and force out the secretion (Plate 14). This prevents any pressure against the globe or trauma to the globe. The expressed material is removed with a cotton-tipped applicator. Each gland in the lower lid is expressed in this fashion. The meibomian glands of the upper lid can be expressed in a similar fashion. The patient is instructed to look down and the upper lid is lifted away from the globe and the cotton-tipped applicator is placed under the lid and held against the tarsal conjunctiva. Pressure is applied with the thumb to the lid and the glands are expressed. In-office gland expression should be done every 4–6 weeks until lid hygiene at home is sufficient to keep the glands expressed.

In addition to the in-office procedure, or in place of it for mild to moderate cases, home lid hygiene is necessary. This should consist of warm compresses two to four times per day followed by lid scrubs and massage. The patient is instructed to heat a wash cloth under hot water. The wash cloth should be as hot as the patient can easily tolerate. The cloth is then held against the closed eye until the cloth begins to cool and then it is heated again. This is repeated such that the hot compress is in place a total of 5–10 minutes. The hot compresses both soften (melt) the sebum in the meibomian glands and the debris at the base of the lashes if there is a blepharitis. The normal lipids from the meibomian glands begin to melt at 32°C, whereas the lipids from abnormal glands do not begin to melt until the temperature has reached 35°C.[98]

After the hot compresses have been applied, the patient should scrub the lids. This can be done by using the warm, wetted wash cloth alone to scrub the lid margin using horizontal strokes. Baby shampoo, either full strength or diluted 50%, can be used on the wash cloth to enhance the cleaning effect. Commercially prepared lid scrubs are available and also work well. The important aspect is the mechanical rubbing effect. It is important to both remove the debris from the base of the lashes and to massage the lid to express the glands. In addition to the lid scrubs the patient can be instructed to massage the lids by placing the index finger on the lid just outside the lashes and pressing gently against the globe working in a circular fashion toward the lid margin. This should be done along the entire extent of both the lower and upper lid.

Korb and Greiner found marked symptomatic relief, less solidified sebum, a significant increase in tear film lipid layer thickness, and a more stable tear film after 6 months of in-office expression every 6 weeks and daily use of warm compresses and lid scrubs.[97]

If staphylococcal blepharitis is present, a topical antibiotic may be used. Bacitracin is usually the drug of first choice and is generally selected empirically without cultures, since in most cases it is effective and has a low incidence of sensitivity reactions. If this medication is not effective, specimens for culture should be taken after at least 24–48 hours of no treatment. Erythromycin is the second most commonly used medication. It is used in an ointment form, which is applied to the lid margins at the base of the lashes by rubbing it in place with either the tip of the finger or a cotton-tipped swab after the lid scrubs. This should be done after each lid hygiene session (two to four times a day) until the infection is brought under control. The patient can also be placed on nonpreserved artificial tears every 2–4 hours. The goal is to discontinue the medication and control the condition with lid scrubs only.

Steroid therapy is not usually necessary or prudent in most cases unless the condition is severe and is causing infiltration and neovascularization of the cornea.

The warm compresses, lid scrubs, and massage should be done two to four times per day for 2 weeks to 3 months or until the lids and glands have improved. This should be done in the morning not long after awakening to remove material that has built up overnight and then at least again before retiring in the evening. It must be remembered, and the patient informed, that this is a chronic condition and once the acute therapy is completed the patient must continue to do the lid hygiene once a day to once a week depending on the patient to maintain adequate gland function. The patient should perform the above procedures in the office to be sure they know how and can perform the lid hygiene properly.

Patients with grade 3 or grade 4 meibomian gland dysfunction can be put on oral tetracycline or doxycycline in addition to the above therapy. The typical tetracycline dose is 250 mg four times a day, taken on an empty stomach, until the dysfunction is under control and then the dosage is tapered down over 4–12 weeks. The reason that this therapy works is not known but it may reduce the bacteria present and thus the lipolytic enzymes they produce.[99] Tetracycline does have adverse effects. It can cause nausea and gastritis. It has photosensitizing properties; therefore, the patient should avoid exposure to sunlight. It should not be given to children or during pregnancy or when breast feeding. Erythromycin is an acceptable alternative when required. Doxycycline is given in a dosage of 100 mg twice a day for 2–4 weeks.

Summary of Treatment of Meibomian Gland Dysfunction and Blepharitis

1. Hot compresses two to four times per day
2. Lid scrubs two to four times per day
3. Massage of the lids after lid scrubs if there is meibomian gland dysfunction
4. Expression of the meibomian glands (if there is severe meibomian gland dysfunction) every 4–6 weeks in the practitioner's office for 6 months
5. Topical bacitracin ointment (if there is blepharitis) applied after each lid scrub
6. Tetracycline 250 mg PO qid for 2–4 weeks and tapered over 4–12 weeks (if there is meibomian gland dysfunction)

Nutrition and Nutritional Supplements

It is well known that malnutrition results in dry eye. A decrease in protein and vitamin A intake can have devastating effects. The effect of dietary supplementation on the tear film for individuals with apparently adequate diets is controversial and has recently been receiving attention. In a comprehensive review of the effect of diet on tear function, Caffery has indicated that deficiencies in vitamins A,

B_6, and C, minerals (potassium, zinc), folate, and linoleic acid may be involved in tear dysfunction.[100] Patel et al. found that a supplement of a multiple vitamin and trace element tablet as well as a pure vitamin C tablet increased the tear thinning time significantly compared with a control group of patients.[101, 102]

Alcohol and caffeine can cause dehydration and may accentuate dry-eye problems. Increasing water intake may help patients with dry-eye symptoms.

Although there is a lack of sufficient scientific studies to unequivocally show an effect of diet on tear function, the literature suggests that there may be an effect. Caffery[100] has suggested the following dietary advice for those with tear film problems:

1. Balance the intake of macronutrients by lowering protein, total fat, and cholesterol and increasing the intake of complex carbohydrates.
2. Increase vitamin A intake (red, orange, yellow, and dark green vegetables).
3. Increase zinc and folate intake (whole grains, legumes, raw vegetables).
4. Ensure sufficient vitamin B_6 and potassium intake (nuts, bananas, beans).
5. Ensure sufficient vitamin C intake (citrus fruit).
6. Eliminate alcohol and caffeine.
7. Increase water intake.

Material Properties

As discussed earlier, lenses of higher water content tend to lose more water than low water content lenses. In addition to the effect of water content, it would be helpful to know if there is any difference in dehydration rates of different materials of the same water content.

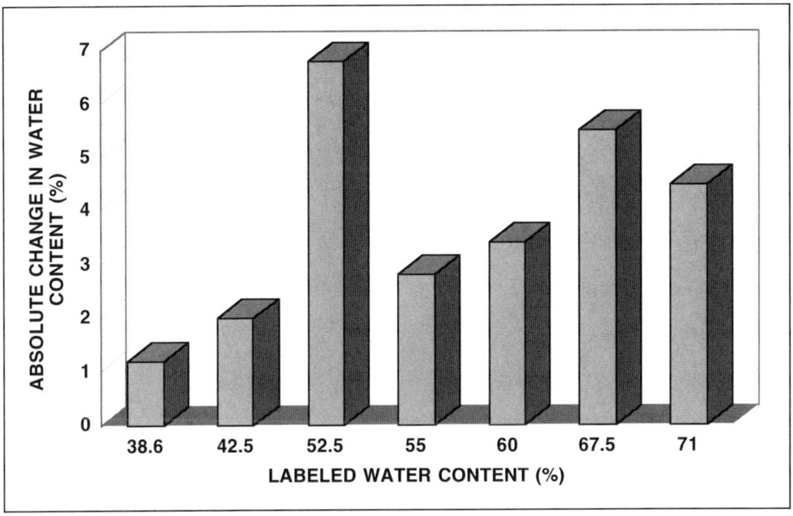

FIGURE 25. Dehydration of different water content hydrogel materials with lens wear. (Modified with permission from NA Brennan, N Efron. Hydrogel lens dehydration: a material-dependent phenomenon? Contact Lens Forum 1987;April 28–29, pp 28–29.)

Are there any differences resulting from manufacturing technique—for example, between lathe cut, spun cast, and molded lenses?

In one study where the in vivo water content was measured, there was the generally expected trend that as the fully hydrated lens water content increased, the amount of water lost increased (Figure 25).[103] There were exceptions, however. A 52.5% water content lens lost more water than the 60–71% water content lenses tested. This indicates that although the general trend is for more loss of water with higher water contents, there is a material or manufacturing difference that may be important.

In another in vivo study, Acuvue (Vistakon, Inc.) lenses lost 6.2% of their water in 20 minutes of wear and 10.2% after 6 hours of wear.[104] This water loss was greater than reported with other lenses of similar water content, again indicating a difference with material.

Mackie measured the loss in weight of different thickness hydrogel lenses and found that the rate of water loss was the same regard-

Table 14. U.S. Food and Drug Administration Lens Classifications

Group	*Water Content*	*Charge*
I	<50%	Nonionic
II	>50%	Nonionic
III	<50%	Ionic
IV	>50%	Ionic

less of starting thickness.[105] This held true for 78%, 55%, and 38% water content lenses. This would be expected since the water is being lost from the surface; thus, for a given water content material with the same surface area, the same amount of water would be lost. The percentage of water lost from the thin lens would be more since there is less total water present. Mackie did find a greater water loss from the high water content lens than from the low water content lens, confirming previous findings that high water content lenses in general dehydrate faster.

Helton and Watson determined the rate of dehydration in air (not on the eye) of various lenses by measuring the weight loss of the lenses.[106] They studied 11 different lenses with water contents ranging from 38% to 74%. They compared a number of different lens groups. One comparison was between the four U.S. Food and Drug Administration lens categories (Table 14). They did not find a significant difference between groups II, III, and IV. However, there was a significant difference between group I lenses and the other groups (Figure 26). One limitation of this study was that only one group III lens (DuraSoft 2, Wesley-Jesson, Inc.) was tested. Since group I and group III lenses have the same water content, one would expect them to dehydrate at similar rates. These results suggest that the ionic nature of the material may be a factor. Another interesting finding was that SeeQuence (Bausch and Lomb) lenses dehydrated more rapidly than other group I lenses. Likewise, in comparing Acuvue and NewVue (Ciba Vision Care) disposable lenses to other group IV lenses, the Acuvue lenses dehydrated the

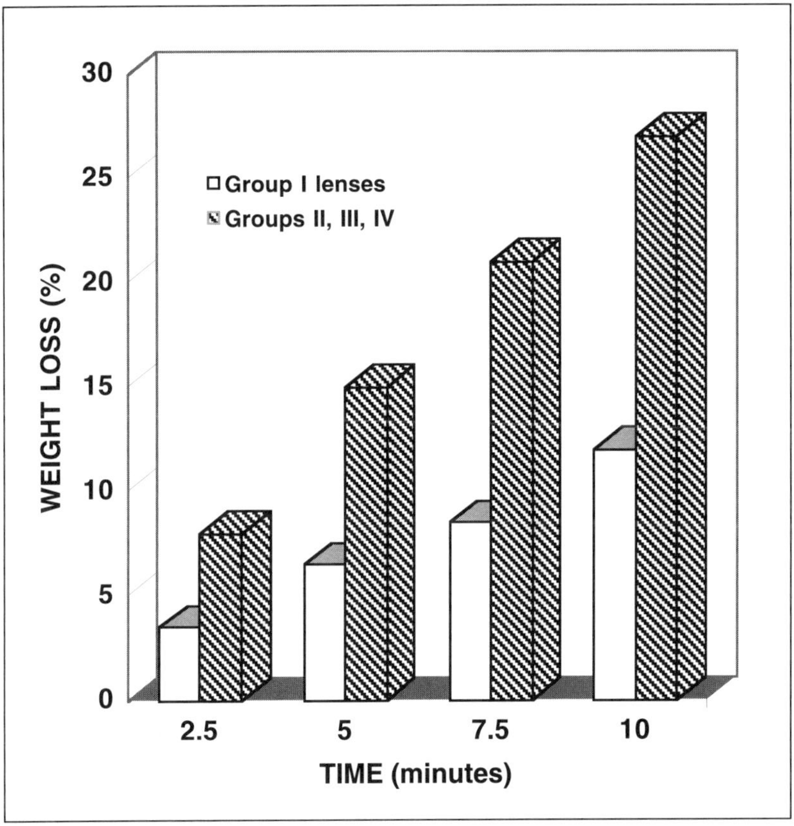

FIGURE 26. Dehydration of group I hydrogel lenses versus other groups of lenses. Note the lower rate of dehydration for group I lenses. (Modified with permission from DO Helton, LS Watson. Hydrogel contact lens dehydration rates determined by thermogravimetric analysis. CLAO J 1991;17:59.)

most, followed by other group IV lenses with the NewVue lenses dehydrating the least (Figure 27). The lens thickness and weight have an effect on the rate of water loss and these factors were not necessarily controlled in this study.

Anderson and Lowther measured the dehydration rates of various lenses using an electronic balance interfaced with a computer to record the weight loss over time.[107] The rate of dehydration was very consistent for a given lens type. When comparing a spun-cast

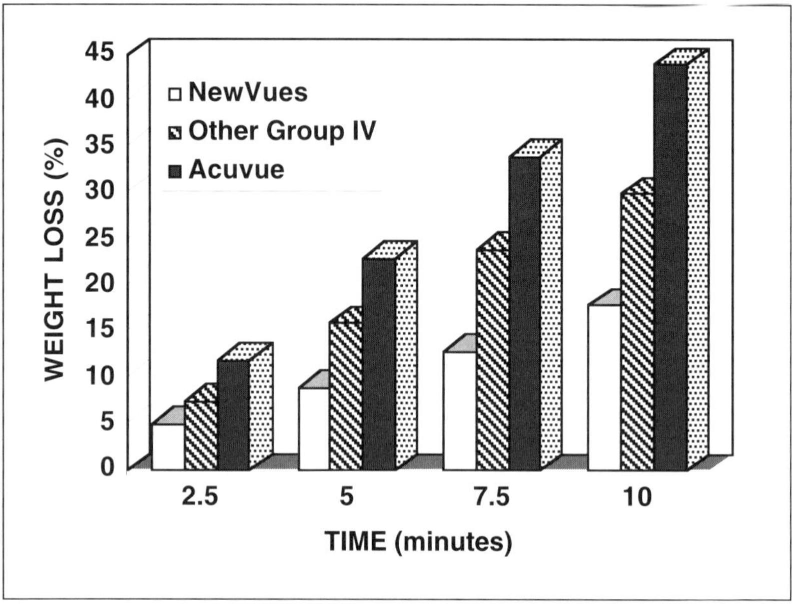

FIGURE 27. Dehydration rates of NewVue and Acuvue lenses versus other group IV lenses. (Modified with permission from DO Helton, LS Watson. Hydrogel contact lens dehydration rates determined by thermogravimetric analysis. CLAO J 1991;17:59.)

lens with the front surface formed against a mold and back against air (SeeQuence) versus a spun-cast front with a lathe-cut back surface (SeeQuence 2) there was some difference in dehydration rates beyond 20 minutes (Figure 28). The SeeQuence 2 had a greater initial weight, and the curves in Figure 28 are normalized to the same weight to illustrate the dehydration differences. The small difference beyond 20 minutes is probably not clinically important. Comparing four different materials of essentially the same labeled water content (55%) and center thickness (0.05–0.07 mm), it can be seen that the Acuvue, NewVue, and DuraSoft 3 lenses all dehydrated at approximately the same rate (Figure 29). This is not consistent with the findings of Helton and Watson.[106] The Softmate 2 (Pilkington Barnes Hind) dehydrated at a greater rate than the others; however, its initial weight was considerably greater. All

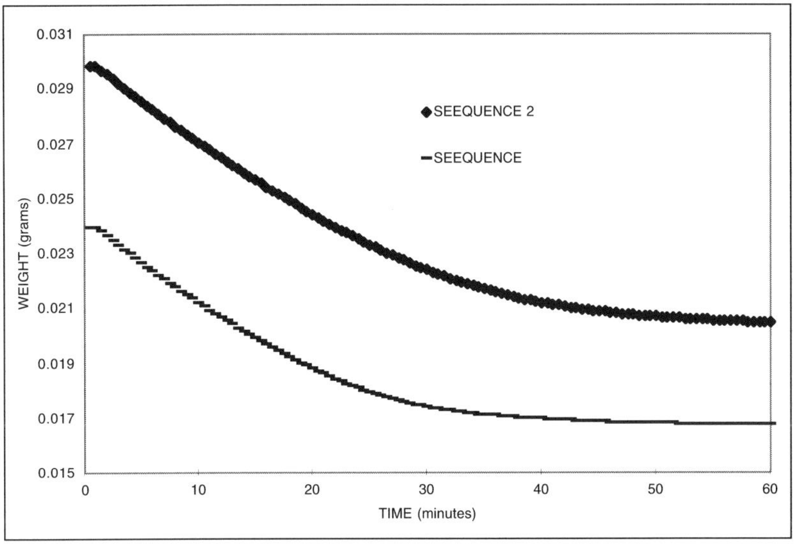

FIGURE 28. Dehydration rate of a spun-cast lens (SeeQuence) versus a spun-cast lens with a lathe-cut back surface (SeeQuence 2). Each curve is the mean of measurements of six –4.00 D lenses. The curves were normalized to the same initial weight for comparison of dehydration rates. (Data from J Anderson, GE Lowther. Dehydration Rates of Selected Hydrogel Lenses. Presented as a poster at the B&L Contact Lens Research Symposium, San Diego, August 1993.)

were –4.00 D lenses. When three lenses (CSI [Pilkington Barnes Hind], CibaSoft [Ciba Vision Care], DuraSoft 2) of the same water content, power, and center thickness but different polymers were compared, it was found that the CSI lens dehydrated at a different rate than the other two lenses (Figure 30). This again indicates that different polymers do dehydrate at different rates. The impression is that CSI lenses seem to cause more "smile" staining (inferior mid-periphery staining) than other lens types. This is possibly a result of the dehydration rate.

Another concern is the effect of tints on dehydration rates. Figure 31 shows the dehydration in air of two identical lenses except one has a blue tint. As can be seen for this particular tint and tinting process, there was no difference in the rate of water loss. In com-

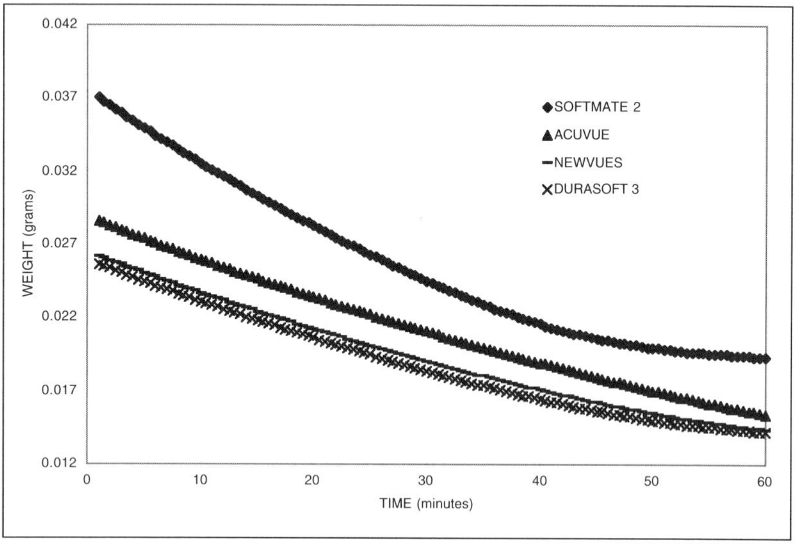

FIGURE 29. Comparison of the dehydration rates in air of some group IV lenses. All the lenses dehydrated at approximately the same rate. Each curve is the mean of measurements of six −4.00 D lenses. (Data from J Anderson, GE Lowther. Dehydration Rates of Selected Hydrogel Lenses. Presented as a poster at the B&L Contact Lens Research Symposium, San Diego, August 1993.)

paring DuraSoft 3 clear and opaque tints, there was a difference (Figure 32). The opaque lens had a greater initial thickness but appeared to dehydrate more rapidly than the clear lens.

What We Know About the Effect of Material on Dehydration

1. Group I lenses appear to dehydrate slower.
2. There appear to be differences in dehydration rates within a group.
3. Transparent tints do not appear to affect dehydration rate.
4. Some opaque lenses appear to have a different dehydration rate than clear lenses.

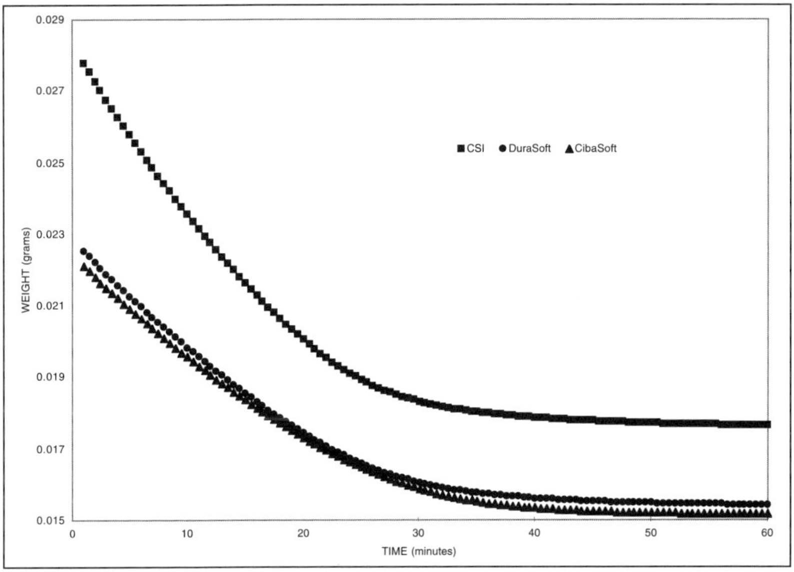

FIGURE 30. Comparison of the dehydration rate in air of three lenses of the same water content showing that there can be differences in dehydration rates. Each curve is the mean of measurements of six –4.00 D lenses. (Data from J Anderson, GE Lowther. Dehydration Rates of Selected Hydrogel Lenses. Presented as a poster at the B&L Contact Lens Research Symposium, San Diego, August 1993.)

Design Considerations

From the work of Andrasko and others we know that high water content lenses and thinner lenses dehydrate most rapidly. Logically from this it would be expected that thicker, low water content lenses would minimize dehydration. The question is, does this hold up in clinical practice?

Finnemore carried out a series of studies designed to test this hypothesis (personal communication). Using 60 patients with symptoms of drying, he fitted one eye with a 0.06-mm–thick, 38% water content lens and the other eye with a 0.12-mm–thick lens. Sixty percent of the patients preferred the thicker lens, 20% the thinner lens, and 20% could not tell a difference. Using 40 of these same patients he fitted one eye with a 0.06-mm, 38% water content lens and the other eye with a 0.15-mm, 50% water content lens. Seventy percent of the patients pre-

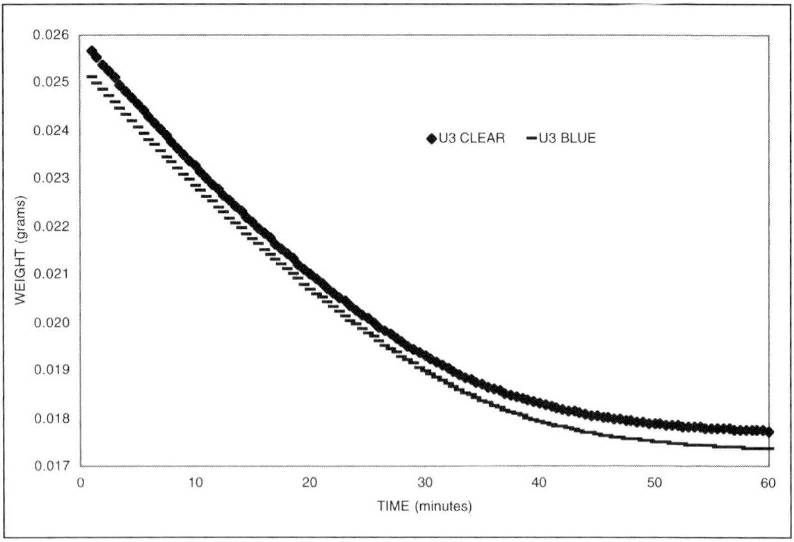

FIGURE 31. Dehydration rate in air of two identical lenses except one is clear and the other has an enhancing tint. Each curve is the mean of measurements of six –4.00 D lenses. (Data from J Anderson, GE Lowther. Dehydration Rates of Selected Hydrogel Lenses. Presented as a poster at the B&L Contact Lens Research Symposium, San Diego, August 1993.)

ferred the thicker, higher water content lens, with 13% of the patients preferring the thin lens and the others finding no difference. In a third experiment he used the same 40 patients with them wearing the lens they preferred from the previous study on one eye and a 38% water content prism-ballasted lens on the opposite eye. In this case 73% of the patients preferred the prism-ballasted lens and 15% the spherical lens. From this study it appears that the thicker the lens the fewer the drying symptoms. It is not known if the prism ballasted lens was preferred just because it was thicker in the more exposed part of the eye or if there was some other effect caused by the design. The question of the water content in the clinical situation is still not answered. What would happen with two identical lenses with respect to thickness, for example 0.15 mm, but different water contents, such as 38% and 55%?

In a retrospective study of 54 patients diagnosed with dry eye who were fitted with contact lenses, 61% were successful.[108] The

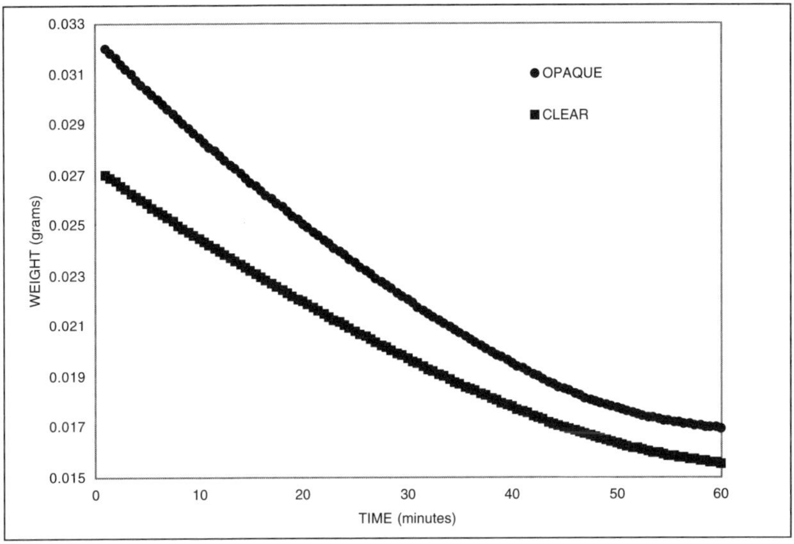

FIGURE 32. Dehydration rate in air of two identical lenses (DuraSoft 3) except one is clear and the other has an opaque tint. Each curve is the mean of measurements of six –4.00 D lenses. (Data from J Anderson, GE Lowther. Dehydration Rates of Selected Hydrogel Lenses. Presented as a poster at the B&L Contact Lens Research Symposium, San Diego, August 1993.)

greatest number of the patients were successful with low water content lenses (74% versus 19% with medium and 7% with high water content lenses). The authors also concluded that thin lenses (0.06–0.10 mm) were more successful, but since it was a retrospective study, there was insufficient information to determine the correlation between thickness and water content.

What We Know About Lens Design and Dryness

1. Thick lenses seem to be preferred.
2. Prism-ballasted lenses may perform better than spherical lenses.
3. Low water content is probably better than high water content.

Use of Punctal Plugs

Since dehydration of hydrogel lenses and the loss of tear volume may be part of the cause of the signs and symptoms of dryness, methods to increase or maintain the tear volume on the eye are logical approaches to solving the problem. One way to maintain more tear volume on the eye would be to prevent loss of tears from the eye via the drainage system. Since excess tears are drained through the puncta to the canaliculi into the lacrimal sac and then into the nasal cavity, closing either the puncta or the canaliculi would prevent tear loss by this route. The other two ways tears are lost from the surface of the eye, evaporation and reabsorption into the conjunctiva, would remain. Milder estimated that 10–25% of the tears are lost by evaporation under normal conditions.[109] Mathers and Daley found that 29% of the tears are lost by evaporation in normal subjects and 69% of the tears are lost by this route in patients with lacrimal insufficiency.[110]

It is important to understand how the tears are drained through the system. The tears only flow through the puncta with a blink. During a blink the medial portion of the upper and lower lids at the puncta meet first during the lid closure phase and the puncta are sealed.[111, 112] With the puncta closed, the canaliculi are squeezed by the action of the surrounding muscles, forcing the tears into the lacrimal sac.[109] Once the tears are in the lacrimal sac they are either absorbed[113] or drain into the nasolacrimal duct, which drains into the inferior meatus of the nose. When the lids open, the last place where the lids are touching is at the medial portion of the puncta. When the lids finally separate at this point, they "pop" open because of the partial vacuum in the canaliculi.[111] This vacuum effect pulls tears into the puncta; this is why tears and debris are seen in the tear prism along the lid margin flowing toward the puncta just after a blink but not during a period of nonblinking. It is estimated that this drainage system is capable of draining 100 times more tears than needed under normal circumstances.[113]

There has been controversy over the relative roles of the upper versus lower canaliculi in tear drainage. However, recent studies of flow

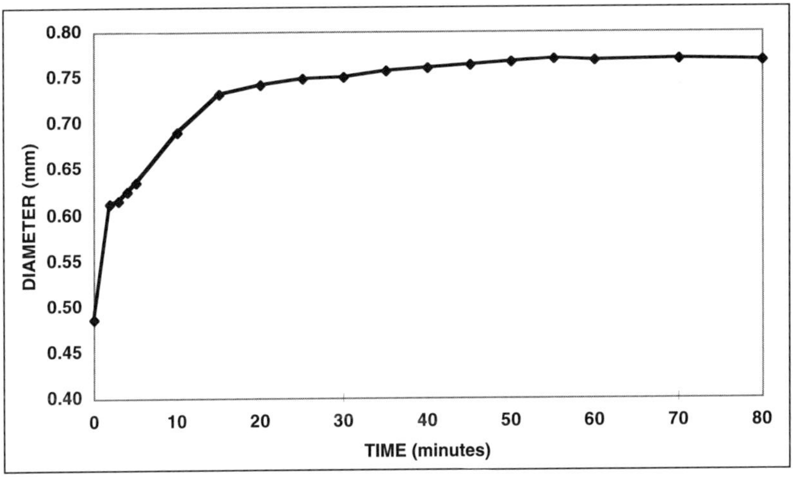

FIGURE 33. The rate of swelling of a collagen implant in vitro in saline solution.

rates by conduction time,[114] dacryoscintigraphy,[115] and fluorescein disappearance[116] all indicate that the upper and lower canaliculi are equal in the drainage of the tears. Because of the vacuum mechanism pulling tears into the canaliculi, an equal contribution of the two would be expected. Plugging only one canaliculus is usually not sufficient to produce any significant effect on tear drainage.[117] Therefore, to be effective in most cases both the upper and lower canaliculi must be closed.

There are a number of ways the puncta and canaliculi can be closed. Collagen implants, which are small rods of collagen (Plate 15), can be placed through the punctum into the canaliculus. These implants come in different diameters (0.2 mm, 0.3 mm, and 0.4 mm) and are approximately 1.5 mm long. They dissolve over time; the manufacturers indicate it takes 5–7 days. However, a recent study has indicated that by 48 hours there is no measurable reduction in outflow with the collagen implants.[118] These collagen implants swell when placed in the canaliculus or in solution. They swell to approximately two times their original diameter in approximately in 30–90 minutes (Figure 33). The potential use of the collagen implants is as a diagnostic test to determine if permanent closure would be effec-

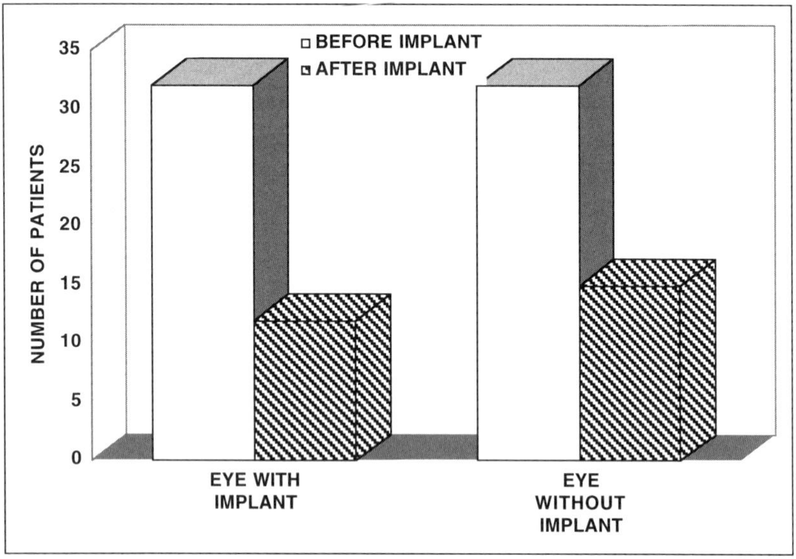

FIGURE 34. Effect of collagen implants on the symptom of dryness with 32 symptomatic patients who had the collagen implants placed in the canalicula of one eye only. (Adapted from GE Lowther, L Semes. Effect of absorbable intracanalicular collagen implants in hydrogel contact lens patients with drying symptoms. ICLC 1995;22:238.)

tive. In a double-masked prospective study of 32 hydrogel lens patients with symptoms of dryness, both canaliculi of one eye of the patients were plugged with a single collagen implant.[119] A sham procedure of placing the implants was done on the other eye, and the patient did not know in which eye the the implants were placed. A number of tests were performed and a questionnaire was filled out by the patients before insertion of the implants and then 5 days afterward. All the patients had the symptom of dryness on entering the study, whereas after the implants were placed only 12 reported dryness in the eye with the implant (Figure 34). However, only 15 of the patients reported the symptom in the eye that did not receive the implants. Similar results were found for the symptoms of burning and grittiness. No significant differences were found with respect to tear prism height, BUT, fluorescein staining, or Lactoplate results between the two eyes. Thus, it was concluded that the implants were not an effective method of determining if permanent closure would be effective. The placebo effect appeared to be very important and misleading in this case. The fact that they were not effective is not surprising knowing the results of the study of Groves et al., which indicated that the average reduction in outflow with the implants was only 16.5% that in normal subjects.[120] Apte found reductions in outflow of 14%, 27%, and 44% in three subjects with dry eyes 2 days after implantation.[121]

Another method for reducing outflow is to use permanent silicone plugs. One plug design, the Freeman Punctal Plug, is such that it fits into the punctum with a small dome being visible in the punctum. These plugs are available in four sizes (0.5 mm, 0.6 mm, 0.7 mm, and 0.8 mm in diameter) and are made of a soft silicone (available from Eagle Vision, Memphis, TN, 800-222-7584). The plug is put into place by pushing the plug down in the punctum. The plug has a hole in the top center and is on a wire holder that is used to manipulate it. Once the plug is in the punctum, the holder is removed and the plug stays in place. It is helpful to dilate the punctum with a punctal dilator before plug insertion. If it is necessary to remove the plug, a small pair of forceps can be used to grasp the plug just below the dome; the plug is then lifted upward while it is slightly tilted at the same time.

Another method for permanently plugging the system is to use the Herrick Lacrimal Plug, which is a small tapered silicone plug. It comes in shaft diameters of either 0.3 mm or 0.5 mm and has a flange ("collapsible bell") that is 0.7 mm or 1.6 mm in diameter, respectively (Figure 35) (available from Lacrimedics, Inc., Rialto, CA, 800-367-8327). The plug comes on a small wire holder that is used to insert it. This plug is placed down into the canaliculus. To place it, the shaft is put into the punctum while it is being held at a 90-degree angle to the lid margin (Plate 16). Once in the punctum, the wire holder is tilted such that it is approximately parallel to the lid margin (Plate 17) and pushed into the canaliculus, which runs nasally parallel to the lid margin. The plug is then pushed through the punctum

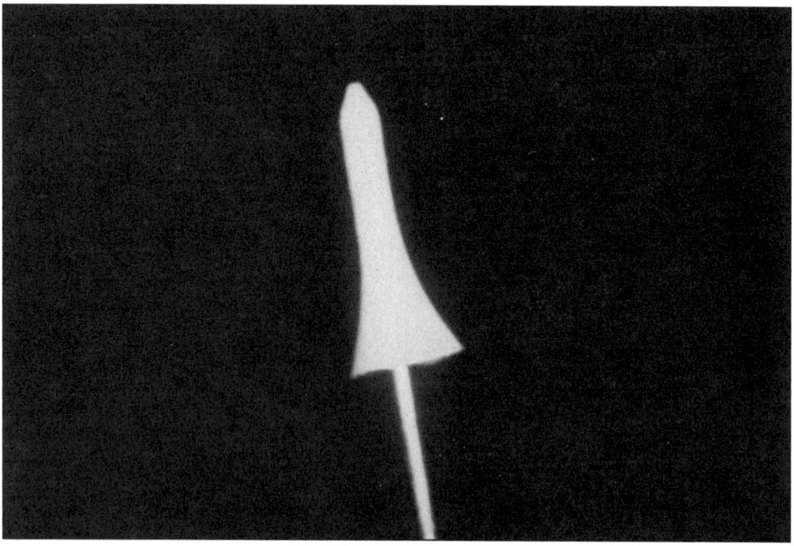

FIGURE 35. A soft silicone Herrick Lacrimal Plug.

into the canaliculus. Once the bell of the plug goes through the punctum, the wire is pulled back out leaving the plug in place. An advantage of this type of plug is that it cannot be seen by the patient or cause any conjunctival or corneal irritation. The disadvantages, compared with the other design of punctal plug, are that you cannot be sure that it is still in place at a later date, and to be removed it must be flushed on through the lacrimal drainage system using lacrimal irrigation. Removing it with lacrimal irrigation is not difficult. A lacrimal dilator attached to a syringe filled with saline is placed into the punctum, first at a 90-degree angle to the lid and then tilted to be approximately parallel to the lid as described for placing the plug. Once the dilator is in place, the saline is forced through the canaliculus, washing the plug into the nasal cavity. If the plug is in place, there will be initial resistance that will require moderate pressure on the syringe to get the saline to flow.

The question is "Does the use of these silicone plugs increase the comfort and decrease the signs of dryness with contact lens wear?"

In one study, Freeman Punctum Plugs (Eagle Vision) were placed in 30 hydrogel lens patients with dryness symptoms.[122] The plugs were placed in the lower punctum of one eye. The invesitgators were not able to place the plugs in five patients, and the plugs had to be removed in another four patients because of irritation. Of the 21 patients who had the plugs in place at the 3-week visit, 18 reported an average 34.6% increase in comfortable wearing time. All 21 patients reported some mild irritation for an average of 1.8 days after plug placement, which prevented masking of the patient as to which eye was plugged.

Slusser used the Herrick plugs on 35 hydrogel patients with symptoms of dryness in a double-masked, placebo-controlled study design.[58] The patients' baseline symptoms, noninvasive BUT, extent of fluorescein and rose bengal staining, and lens water content were measured. The patients filled out a questionnaire about lens dryness, lens awareness, and vision with the lens using a subjective linear scale for each eye for 1 week before entering the study. After the 1 week baseline questionnaire was completed, another examination was performed and the implants were placed in both canaliculi of one eye with the same procedure being performed on the other eye but with no plugs inserted. Therefore, the patient did not know in which eye the plugs were placed. The patients filled out the questionnaires and were examined after 1 and 4 weeks for a period of 4 weeks. During the fifth week with the plugs the patients were instructed to use rewetting drops (Lens Plus Rewetting Drops, Allergan, Inc.) four times a day in each eye. They were asked to not use drops before this last week. Twenty-eight patients completed the study because the plugs could not be inserted in the upper canaliculus of three patients, three patients had the plugs removed because of epiphora, and one patient was not able to return for all the visits. A significant decrease in the symptoms of dryness (Figure 36) and lens awareness in the eye with the plugs versus the eye in which only the sham procedure had been performed was found. There was also a significant decrease of these

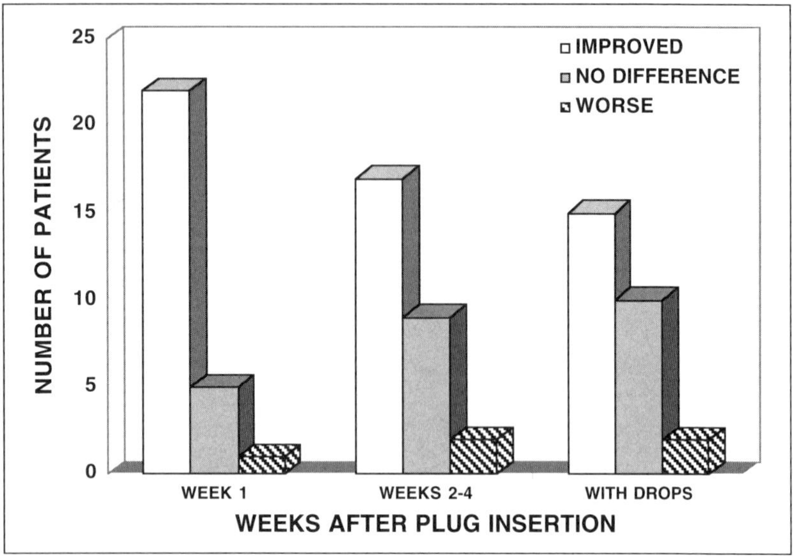

FIGURE 36. Number of contact lens patients (total 28) who reported improvement, no difference, or worsening of dryness symptoms in the eye with a plug versus the control eye after the placement of a Herrick plug in the canaliculi of one eye. (Redrawn with permission from TG Slusser. Effects of Lacrimal Drainage Occlusion with Non-Dissolvable Intracanalicular Plugs on Hydrogel Contact Lens Related Dry Eye. Master of Science Thesis, University of Alabama at Birmingham, 1994.)

symptoms between the baseline measurements and after the plugs were inserted for *both* eyes. There also seemed to be a decrease in the effectiveness of the plugs over time for some patients. After 1 week, 22 of the patients indicated that the plugged eye was better, 17 indicated it was better during weeks 2–4, and 15 indicated it was better during week 5 (see Figure 36). There may be a feedback system that causes less tears to be produced when there is a surplus of tears present. Another finding that suggests such an adaptation is that 82% of the patients experienced epiphora only during the first few days after insertion of the plugs. Norn has found a decrease in tear production with impaired lacrimal drainage.[123] The question yet to be answered is would this trend continue such that over several months the effect of having the plugs in place would be totally lost. There was a significant decrease in the fluorescein staining on

Table 15. Ranking of Methods of Handling Lens Dehydration with Hydrogel Lens Wear in a Survey of 310 Practitioners

Method	*Rank*
Rewetting drops	1
Reduced wearing time	2
Nonpreserved products	3
Refit with low water content lenses	4
Refit with RGP lenses	5
Refit with mid-water content lenses	6
Lid scrubs	7
Refit with thicker low water lenses	8

Source: Modified from GN Orsborn, SG Zantos. Practitioner survey: management of dry-eye symptoms in soft lens wearers. CL Spectrum 1989;4(9):23.

the eye with the plugs. Only during the fifth week when rewetting drops were being used was there an increase in the water content of the lenses. At the end of the Slusser study, 76% of the patients elected to have the plugs inserted in the second eye with only 18% requesting the plugs be removed from the test eye. The others elected to just keep the plugs in the test eye only. Thus, a majority of the patients felt that plugs made a significant improvement.

From the limited studies performed to date it appears that permanent plugs can give some relief of dryness symptoms with hydrogel lens wear. However, they certainly do not help all patients and there is still a question of long-term effectiveness.

Summary of Therapy for Dryness with Hydrogel Lenses

In a survey of 310 practitioners, it was found that the number one recommendation for patients with drying symptoms with hydrogel lenses was to use rewetting drops. The number two recommendation was to reduce wearing time. A variety of other techniques were commonly recommended (Table 15).[2] From the studies done to date, the management scheme shown in Figure 37 is recommended.

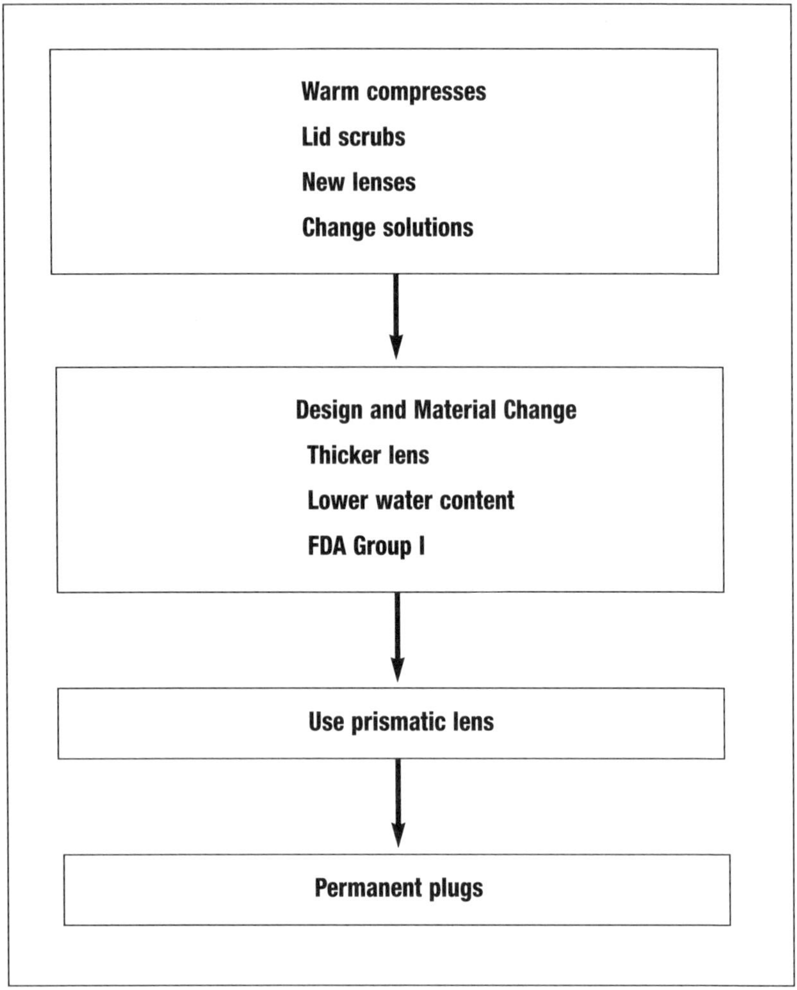

FIGURE 37. Flow chart for the management of patients using hydrogel lenses with symptoms of dryness.

If the lenses are conventional lenses with any deposits they should be replaced, since deposits will cause a short BUT on the lens surface and increase symptoms. You may want to put the patient on unpreserved solutions, as some patients report dryness symptoms are diminished or alleviated with the elimination of preservatives.

Since meibomianitis and blepharitis are so common with contact lens wear, it is recommended that the patient use warm compresses at least twice daily as well as do lid scrubs after the warm compresses. The patient must be given specific instructions for these procedures. The warm compresses should be done first, since the mechanical action of the lid scrubs will not only help remove the debris from the lashes but also will help express the abnormal sebum from the meibomian glands, which will be softened by the warm compresses.

Using a low water content group I lens that is relatively thick, 0.10 mm or greater, often decreases the symptoms. Lenses such as the AMSoft Standard, Aquaflex Standard, Ciba Standard, B&L B3/B4, Hydron Mini-Lens, or other similarly thick lenses can be used. Lenses may have to be fitted flatter than normal, since with dehydration the lens movement may decrease. If all of the above approaches do not sufficiently improve the situation, a prism-ballasted lens may be tried. Permanent plugs can be used as the final attempt to obtain comfortable wear.

Obviously, as in any clinical condition, patients react differently and a given procedure does not work the same on all patients. Whereas low water content lenses seem to work best on most patients, in some cases higher water content lenses are preferred. Lens materials that resist dehydration may be developed, which could decrease dryness problems. As we learn more about dryness and the tear film, the above recommendations may change.

Rigid Gas-Permeable Contact Lenses and Tear Problems

Surface Drying

A common problem with rigid gas-permeable (RGP) lens wear is surface drying between blinks (Plate 18). The tear film forms over the surface of a rigid lens; however, no anterior lipid layer is found on rigid lenses.[19] Without a lipid layer, the exposed aqueous film evaporates at a greater rate than the normal tear film over the cornea. The anterior surface drying time (time from a blink to the formation of a haze on the surface) on polymethylmethacrylate (PMMA) lenses was found to be approximately 4.4–4.8 seconds.[19] With silicone/acrylate lenses the time was found to average 1.77 seconds, whereas with fluorosilicone/acrylate lenses the average time was 3.7 seconds.[124] The surface chemistry of the gas-permeable lenses probably contributes to the more rapid drying. Silicone groups on the lens surface are hydrophobic and thus attract and hold hydrophobic materials such as lipids from the tear film. When there are areas of hydrophobic material on the surface, these areas tend to repel water, like wax on a car, and shorten the time after a blink before the haze occurs. There are compounds added to RGP lenses to attempt to overcome the nonwetting properties of silicone. Compounds such as methylacrylic acid and HEMA are used. These compounds attract and hold charged molecules such as water. The attraction of water is desired to maintain the wettability, but these compounds will also cause charged areas of proteins to attach. The proteins can build up and denature on the surface also causing nonwetting. In some cases the fluorosilicone/acrylate lenses seem to do somewhat better with respect to wettability because of the fluorine.

During the manufacturing of the plastic rods or buttons, there can be changes that cause lens wetting problems. If the material is not mixed properly or is not formed under the correct conditions, the properties can change. Also, during the polishing of the lens surface, if too much heat is built up, the surface may become less wettable.

Since tear film components build up on a lens surface, it is important that the patient clean the surface well after each wearing period. Cleaners with abrasive particles often work well. Cleaning with the abrasive cleaners that is too aggressive can decrease the lens thickness and increase the minus power.[125–128] The tear film components can build up on the inside of the lens also. It is more difficult for the patient to clean the inside surface. With a heavy build-up on the inside of the lens (Plate 19), the lens can become uncomfortable and cause corneal staining (Plate 20). The lens should be dried and inspected under 10–20× magnification, where the coating often looks like an old, cracked varnished surface. By holding the lens up at arm's length toward a light, the coated lens will look hazy. This coating can be quite difficult to remove. Usually it can be removed by diligent rubbing of the inside of the lens with a cotton-tipped applicator and contact lens polish or abrasive cleaner. To prevent it from returning the patient should be instructed to clean the inside of the lens once or twice a week with his or her cleaner and a cotton-tipped applicator.

Lipid materials such as hand creams and cosmetics can get on the lens surface preventing the tear film from forming and causing non-wetting. These can also be difficult to remove with many cleaners. Using a cleaner with alcohol added (for example, MiraFlow [Ciba Vision Care] for patient or office use; or Boston Laboratory Lens Cleaner [Polymer Technology] for in-office use) is effective in removing these lipids. The alcohol cleaner should be immediately rinsed from the lens after cleaning because leaving a lens in such a cleaner will cause lens distortion.[129]

Peripheral Corneal Staining

Peripheral corneal staining, also called peripheral desiccation or 3 and 9 o'clock staining, is one of the most common problems with rigid lens wear. One author reported 43–70% of the RGP wearers in four different studies had peripheral staining of greater than grade 2 (on a scale of 0–6).[130] Another study found peripheral staining in 28% of the daily wear RGP patients and 63% of the extended-wear patients.[131] Henry et al.[132] reported 53% of the patients with extended-wear RGP lenses had peripheral staining. With daily wear lenses the staining may develop over several weeks. With extended-wear, severe peripheral staining can occur within days.

Peripheral corneal staining is seen beyond the edge of the lens and not under the lens. It is not seen where the lens normally moves over the cornea with a blink or eye movements. It is caused by a disruption of the tear film resulting in drying of the tissue with breakdown of the epithelial cells and staining. The tear film disruption can be caused by a lack of wiping of the mucoid layer of the tear film over this peripheral portion of the cornea. The mucoid layer is produced by the goblet cells and mechanically spread over the cornea to produce a hydrophilic surface on the epithelial cells on which the aqueous and lipid layers can form. If the edge of a contact lens is too thick or the edge clearance is too great, the upper lid will bridge over the area between the lens edge and the limbus, leaving an area that is not wiped by the lid. A partial or incomplete blink will also prevent wiping of this area, which will cause drying that results in staining. Thus, a patient may have plenty of tear production with all the tear film components present but still have peripheral staining because of a lack of wiping of the area by the lid. It must be remembered that this staining is not caused by physical trauma of the lens edge hitting this area of the cornea.

Surprisingly most patients have no symptoms with peripheral staining even when quite severe. The most common patient complaint or remark is that their eyes appear red and injected.

The staining may be a slight stippling of the peripheral cornea or it may progress to a dense, ulcerated area and scarring. Peripheral staining can be classified on a 0–4 scale as indicated in Table 16.

Grade 1 peripheral staining (Plate 21) is not a problem, and the patient can continue to wear the lenses without restrictions except

Table 16. Grading Scale for Peripheral Corneal Staining

Grade	*Description*
0 (none)	No staining present
1 (slight)	A few scattered spots of stippling
2 (mild)	Heavy stippling
3 (moderate)	Coalesced, punctate staining—possibly some mild fluorescein seepage into the stroma
4 (severe)	Heavy coalesced staining with fluorescein penetration into the stroma Scarring and/or neovascularization in the staining area Dellen with opacification present or imminent

that routine follow-up examinations at frequent intervals are required to ensure that the condition does not worsen. If the condition is grade 2 or greater, changes should normally be made to decrease the staining. Grade 2 staining may be tolerated if the patient is followed closely.

Numerous things can cause the staining. A common cause is lens positioning. If the lens constantly rides high the staining is seen in the inferior temporal and nasal areas. In this case the lens design must be changed to obtain a better centered lens that moves better with a blink. A lens with either a base curve that is too flat or too much peripheral clearance may be pulled up by the upper lid and held there. The lids should be used to center the lens and the fluorescein pattern evaluated in the centered position to determine if the lens is too flat; if it is, it should be corrected. A high minus lens may be held too high because of the thicker edge and wedge effect created. In this case a front surface bevel or lenticular cut to decrease edge thickness may allow the lens to assume a more centered position. A lens that is too small may also be held up excessively high. Going to a larger lens diameter may result in better centration and more coverage of the cornea, thereby keeping it moist.

If the contact lens rides too low and is not picked up and moved sufficiently with a blink, the staining will be in the superior nasal and temporal areas of the palpebral aperture. This inferior position may also be caused by a lens that has a base curve or periphery that is too flat, allowing the lens to drop down over the limbus and remain in this position. In this case the lid does not have enough tension or does not cover enough of the cornea to hold the lens up. Again, the lens fluorescein pattern should be evaluated in the centered position and if it is too flat, appropriate changes should be made. The lens may also be too small, preventing the upper lid from being able to hold it up. In this case a larger overall diameter is required. If the lens is a low minus or plus it will drop and position low because of the wedge effect of the edge ("watermelon seed effect"). Designing the lens with a minus carrier lenticular portion will allow the upper lid to hold the lens up.

The staining may be caused by a thick lens edge. With a thick edge the upper lid, with its rather stiff tarsal plate, will bridge the area between the edge and the limbus or sclera, preventing wiping of the peripheral region of the cornea. Thinning the edge may eliminate or minimize the problem.

Excessive peripheral clearance can cause the same problem. The excessive edge clearance also causes a large meniscus at the edge of the lens. The fluid in the meniscus draws more water into it by capillary attraction, causing a thinning of the surrounding tear film and further compounding the drying. With high magnification one can see a "black line" just beyond the meniscus where there is minimal fluorescein in the tear film because of this thinning. Using steeper peripheral radii can alleviate this cause.

Excessive edge thickness or clearance can also cause discomfort on blinking. The patient may get in the habit of only partially blinking or inhibiting the blink to decrease the discomfort, thus increasing the drying. Reshaping the edge, decreasing the edge lift, increasing the lens diameter, or all of these approaches to improve comfort can alleviate the staining problem.

A lens that is too steep—either base curve or peripheral curve—can cause peripheral staining. The lens does not move over the peripheral cornea and the lid gap prevents wetting, causing a breakdown of the cells and staining. Refitting the patient with a flatter base curve or peripheral curves to improve movement can alleviate the problem.

Lenses with very large optical zones may cause peripheral staining. The edge of the large optical zone is positioned on a flatter part of the cornea, since the cornea flattens toward the limbus. When the edge of the optical zone impinges on this flat part of the cornea, it prevents the lens from moving over the peripheral cornea, thereby allowing the constantly exposed corneal area to dry.

The lens material may contribute to the staining. Materials that do not wet well may cause the staining as the tear film disrupts on the lens surface, increasing tear film evaporation. Using more wettable materials such as lower Dk or fluorosilicone/acrylate materials may help.

If peripheral staining persists with all rigid lens designs, the patient may have to be refitted with hydrogel lenses that cover this area of the cornea and limbus, thus preventing the desiccation. Other drying symptoms as previously described may, however, be a problem.

Rewetting drops seldom have a significant, long lasting effect on peripheral staining.

Summary of Methods to Alleviate Peripheral Staining

1. Improve centration.
   a. Steepen base curve, peripheral curve, or both, if indicated.
   b. Increase diameter.
   c. Flatten base curve, peripheral curve, or both, if indicated.
   d. Use lenticular cut on high minus lenses to decrease edge thickness and lift.
   e. Use minus carrier lenticular on low riding plus or low minus lenses.

2. Decrease edge thickness.
3. Decrease the optical zone diameter.
4. Increase overall diameter.
5. Use a more wettable material.
6. Refit with a hydrogel lens.

Lens Adherence (Binding)

Lens adherence (no lens movement) is a common phenomenon with rigid extended-wear lenses. Different studies have shown the occurrence on initial awakening to be 22%,[133] 48%,[37] and 49%[134] of cases. It also occurs, although less frequently, with daily RGP lens wear.

The cause of the adherence is thought to be a loss of the aqueous layer from under the lens, which allows the mucoid layer to act as a glue.[38] The decreased tear production during sleep as well as the pressure of the lids forcing fluid from under the lens may cause the adherence. When rigid lenses adhere they often leave an impression ring (Plate 22). This has been reported to occur with 53% of those lenses that adhere.[133] Corneal staining is also common. The adherence is not caused by a negative pressure (suction) effect, since tears (with fluorescein) can be forced under three-fourths of the lens and the lens remains adherent. If it were a suction effect, pumping any fluorescein under the lens would release the pressure and initiate movement.

Adherent lenses are usually decentered nasally, bridging the limbus.[133] None of the adherent lenses were centered. Thus, this problem might be minimized by improving lens centration. It was found that lenses that were fitted steeper than K as well as lenses less than 9.5 mm in diameter and with optimal to excessive movement bound less.

In many cases an adherent lens will spontaneously move sometime after awakening. Movement of bound lenses can be achieved by instilling a couple of drops of rewetting or artificial tear solution and then nudging the edge of the lens with the lid margin and blinking until solution is forced under the entire lens.

Hydrogel Versus Rigid Gas-Permeable Lenses for Dry Eyes

There is always the question of which lens type is best for a marginally or frankly dry eye. There are varying clinical opinions and no studies that give a definitive answer. In practice, patients with dry eyes will have difficulty with both types of lenses. Often patients will have less dryness symptoms with RGP lenses, but peripheral corneal staining and resultant injection are problems. With hydrogel lenses the peripheral staining will be alleviated, but the patient may complain of more symptoms. The best clinical advice at this point is, if drying problems develop with one lens type, do not be afraid to switch to the other type, as the patient may do better with the other lens. When there is a drying problem and you change to the other lens type, be sure to use the lens design in the new lens that will minimize the chances of problems. For example, a low water content, relatively thick hydrogel lens or a larger diameter, minimal edge clearance, well-centered RGP lens with thin edges.

References

1. Orsborn G, Robby M. Hydrogel lenses and dry eye symptoms. J Br Contact Lens Assoc 1989;6:37.
2. Orsborn GN, Zantos SG. Practitioner survey: management of dry-eye symptoms in soft lens wearers. CL Spectrum 1989;4(9):23.
3. Brennan NA, Efron N. Symptomatology of HEMA contact lens wear. Optom Vis Sci 1989;66:834.
4. Hathaway RA, Lowther GE. Factors influencing the rate of deposit formation on hydrophilic lenses. Aust J Optom 1978;61:92.
5. Nilsson SEG, Andersson L. Contact lens wear in dry environments. Acta Ophthalmol 1986;64:221.
6. Andrasko G, Schoessler JP. The effect of humidity on the dehydration of soft contact lenses on the eye. ICLC 1980;7:210.
7. Andrasko G. The amount and time course of soft contact lens dehydration. J Am Optom Assoc 1982;53:207.
8. Wechsler S, Prather DL, Sosnowski JS. In vivo hydration of gel lenses. ICLC 1982;9:154.
9. DeDonato LM. Changes in the hydration of hydrogel contact lenses with wear. Am J Optom Physiol Opt 1982;59:213.
10. Brennan NA, Efron N, Truong VT, Watkins RD. Definitions for hydration changes of hydrogel lenses. Ophthalmic Physiol Opt 1986;6:333.
11. Wechsler S, Johnson MH, Businger U. In vivo hydration of hydrogel lenses—the first hour. ICLC 1983;10:349.
12. Sarver MD, Baggett DA, Harris MG, Louie K. Corneal edema with hydrogel lenses and eye closure: effect of oxygen transmissibility. Am J Optom Physiol Opt 1981;58:386.
13. Paugh JR. Equivalent oxygen percentage as a function of hydration in hydrogel lenses: an in vivo study. Optom Vis Sci 1992;69:805.
14. Kohler JE, Flanagan GW. Clinical dehydration of extended wear lenses. ICLC 1985;12:152.
15. Andrasko G. Hydrogel dehydration in various environments. ICLC 1983;10:22.
16. Brennan NA, Efron N, Bruce AS, et al. Dehydration of hydrogel lenses: environmental influences during normal wear. Am J Optom Physiol Opt 1988;65:277.
17. Guillon JP. Tear film photography and contact lens wear. J Br Contact Lens Assoc 1982;5:84.
18. Korb DR. Tear Film–Contact Lens Interactions. In DA Sullivan (ed), Lacrimal Gland, Tear Film and Dry Eye Syndromes. New York: Plenum, 1994.

19. Guillon JP. Tear Film Structure and Contact Lenses. In F Holly (ed), The Preocular Tear Film in Health, Disease, and Contact Lens Wear. Lubbock, TX: Dry Eye Institute, 1986;914.
20. Korb DR, Herman JP, Exford JM, et al. Tear film lipid layer thickness as a function of blinking. Cornea 1994;13:354.
21. Cedarstaff TH, Tomlinson A. A comparative study of tear evaporation rates and water content of soft contact lenses. Am J Optom 1983;60:167.
22. Monster AW, Chan HC, O'Connor. Long-term trends in human eye blink rate. Biotelemetry Patient Monit 1978;5:206.
23. Luckiesh M. Reading and the rate of blinking. J Exp Psychol 1947;37:266.
24. Carpenter A. The rate of blinking during prolonged visual search. J Exp Psychol 1948;38:587.
25. York M, Ong J, Robbins JC. Variation in blink rate associated with contact lens wear and task difficulty. Am J Optom 1971;48:461.
26. Takano H, Takamura E, Yoshimo K, Tsubota K. The Increase of the Blink Interval in Ophthalmic Procedures. In DA Sullivan (ed), Lacrimal Gland, Tear Film, and Dry Eye Syndromes. New York: Plenum, 1994;525.
27. Tsubota K, Nakamori K. Dry eyes and video display terminals. N Engl J Med 1983;328:584.
28. Yaginuma H, Yamada H, Hagai H. Study of the relationship between lacrimation and blink in VDT work. Ergonomics 1990;33:799.
29. Patel S, Henderson R, Bradley L, et al. Effect of video display unit use on blink rate and tear stability. Optom Vis Sci 1991;68:888.
30. Collins M, Seeto R, Campbell L, Ross M. Blinking and corneal sensitivity. Acta Ophthalmol 1989;67:525.
31. Carney LG, Hill RM. Variation in blinking behavior during soft lens wear. ICLC 1984;11:250.
32. Yolton DP, Yolton RL, Lopez R, et al. The effects of gender and birth control pill use on spontaneous blink rates. J Am Optom Assoc 1994;65:763.
33. Holden BA, Sweeney DF, Seger RG. Epithelial erosions caused by thin high water content lenses. Clin Exp Optom 1986;69:103.
34. Zantos SG, Orsborn GN, Walter HC, Knoll HA. Studies on corneal staining with thin hydrogel contact lenses. J Br Contact Lens Assoc 1986;9:61.
35. Orsborn GN, Zantos SG. Corneal desiccation staining with thin high water content contact lenses. Contact Lens Assoc Ophthal J 1988;14:81.
36. Zadnik K, Mutti DO. Inferior arcuate corneal staining in soft contact lens wearers. ICLC 1985;12:110.
37. Kenyon E, Polse KA, Mandell RB. Rigid contact lens adherence: incidence, severity and recovery. J Am Optom Assoc 1988;59:168.
38. Swarbrick HA. A possible etiology for RGP lens binding (adherence). ICLC 1988;15:13.

39. Bruce AS, Brennan NA. Hydrogel lens binding and the post-lens tear film. Clin Eye Vis Care 1992;4:111.
40. Krupin T, Cross DA, Becker B. Decreased basal tear production associated with general anesthesia. Arch Ophthalmol 1977;95:107.
41. Brennan NA, Lowe R, Efron N, et al. Dehydration of hydrogel lenses during overnight wear. Am J Optom Physiol Opt 1987;64:534.
42. Mishima S. Some physiological aspects of the precorneal tear film. Arch Ophthalmol 1965;73:233.
43. Prydal JI, Campbell FW. Study of tear film thickness and structure by interferometry and confocal microscopy. Invest Ophthalmol Vis Sci 1992;33:1996.
44. Prydal JI, Artal P, Woon H, Campbell FW. Study of human tear film thickness using laser interferometry. Invest Ophthalmol Vis Sci 1992;33:2006.
45. Kaura R. Tiffany JM. The Role of Mucus Glycoproteins in the Tear Film. In FJ Holly (ed), The Precorneal Tear Film. Lubbock, TX: Dry Eye Institute, 1986;728.
46. Schoessler JP, Lowther GE. Cell and tear film debris on the posterior surface of an extended wear lens (photoatlas). ICLC 1979;6:30.
47. Wilson G, O'Leary DJ, Holden BA. Cell content of tears following overnight wear of a contact lens. Curr Eye Res 1989;8:329.
48. Tan KO, Sack RA, Holden BA, Swarbrick HA. Temporal sequence of changes in tear film composition during sleep. Curr Eye Res 1993;12:1001.
49. Madigan MC, Holden BA, Kwok LS. Extended wear of contact lenses can compromise corneal epithelial adhesion. Curr Eye Res 1987;6:1257.
50. Lowther GE. Epithelial lesions with hydrogel extended wear: will disposable lenses prevent the problem. ICLC 1988;15:237.
51. Knop E, Brewitt H. Conjunctival cytology in asymptomatic wearers of soft contact lenses. Graefes Arch Clin Exp Ophthalmol 1992;230:340.
52. Griener JV, Allansmith MR. Effect of contact lens wear on the conjunctival mucous system. Ophthalmology 1981;88:821.
53. Connor CG, Campbell JB, Steel SA, Burke JH. The effects of daily wear contact lenses on goblet cell density. J Am Optom Assoc 1994;65:792.
54. Holly FJ. Diagnosis and treatment of dry eye syndrome. CL Spectrum 1989;4(7):37.
55. McMonnies CW, Ho A. Patient history in screening for dry eye conditions. J Am Optom Assoc 1987;58:296.
56. McMonnies CW, Ho A. Marginal Dry Eye Diagnosis: History Versus Biomicroscopy. In Proceedings of the International Society of Dakryology Symposium, Lubbock, Texas, November 7–10, 1984:32.
57. Lowther GE. Comparison of hydrogel contact lens patients with and without the symptoms of dryness. ICLC 1993;20:191.

58. Slusser TG. Effects of Lacrimal Drainage Occlusion with Non-Dissolvable Intracanalicular Plugs on Hydrogel Contact Lens Related Dry Eye. Master of Science Thesis, University of Alabama at Birmingham, 1994.
59. Bowman RW, Dougherty JM, McCulley JP. Chronic blepharitis and dry eyes. Intl Ophthalmol Clin 1987;27:27.
60. Hom MM, Martinson JR, Knapp LL, Paugh JR. Prevalence of meibomian gland dysfunction. Optom Vis Sci 1990;67:710.
61. Korb DR, Henriquez AS. Meibomian gland dysfunction and contact lens intolerance. J Am Optom Assoc 1980;51:243.
62. McCulley JP, Sciallis GF. Meibomian keratoconjunctivitis oculo-dermal correlates. Contact Lens Assoc Ophthal J 1983;9:130.
63. Caroline PJ, Kame RT. Meibomian Gland Dysfunction. In JA Silbert (ed), Anterior Segment Complications of Contact Lens Wear. New York: Churchill Livingstone, 1994.
64. Robin JB, Noble JR, Suarez E. Meibomian gland evaluation in patients with extended wear soft contact lens deposits. Contact Lens Assoc Ophthal J 1986;12:95.
65. Rapp J, Broich IR. Lipid deposition on worn soft contact lenses. Contact Lens Assoc Ophthal J 1984;10:235.
66. Norn SM. Tear Film Break-up Time: A Review. In FJ Holly (ed), The Preocular Tear Film in Health, Disease, and Contact Lens Wear. Lubbock, TX: Dry Eye Institute, 1986;52.
67. Marquardt R, Stodtmeister R, Christ T. Modification of Tear Film Break-up Time Test for Increased Reliability. In FJ Holly (ed), The Preocular Tear Film in Health, Disease, and Contact Lens Wear. Lubbock, TX: Dry Eye Institute, 1986;57.
68. Lemp MA, Hamill JR Jr. Factors affecting tear film breakup in normal eyes. Arch Ophthalmol 1973;89:103.
69. Rengstorff RH. The precorneal tear film: breakup time and location in normal subjects. Am J Optom Physiol Opt 1974;51:765.
70. Vanley GR, Leopold IH, Gregg TH. Interpretation of tear film breakup. Arch Ophthalmol 1977;95:445.
71. Kline LN, DeLuca TJ. Effect of gel lens wear on the precorneal tear film. ICLC 1975;2:56.
72. Faber E, Golding TR, Lowe R, Brennan NA. Effect of hydrogel lens wear on tear film stability. Optom Vis Sci 1991;68:380.
73. Mengher LS, Bron AJ, Tonge SR, Gilbert DJ. A non-invasive instrument for clinical assessment of the pre-corneal tear film stability. Curr Eye Res 1985;4:1.
74. Tonge SR, Humsaker J, Holly FJ. Non-invasive assessment of tear film break-up time in a group of normal subjects—implications for contact lens wear. J Br Contact Lens Assoc 1991;14:201.

75. Patel S, Murray D, McKenzie A, et al. Effect of fluorescein on the tear film breakup time and tear thinning time. Am J Optom Physiol Opt 1985;62:188.
76. Korb DR, Herman JP. Corneal staining subsequent to sequential fluorescein instillations. J Am Optom Assoc 1979;50:361.
77. Caffery B. Rethink your approach to dry eye. Optom Manag 1994;29 (May):26.
78. Norn NS. Vital staining of cornea and conjunctiva. Acta Ophthalmol 1962;40:389.
79. Norn NS. Dead, degenerate, and living cells in conjunctival fluid and mucous thread. Acta Ophthalmol (Copenh) 1969;47:1102.
80. Feenstra RPG, Tseng SCG. What is actually stained by rose bengal? Arch Ophthalmol 1992;110:984.
81. Norn MS. Lissamine green: vital staining of cornea and conjunctiva. Acta Ophthalmol (Copenh) 1973;51:483.
82. Norn MS. Diagnosis of Dry Eye. In MA Lemp, R Marquardt (eds), The Dry Eye: A Comprehensive Guide. Berlin: Springer-Verlag, 1992.
83. Nelson JD. Impression cytology. Cornea 1988;7:71.
84. Egbert PR, Lauber S, Maurice DM. A simple conjunctival biopsy. Am J Ophthalmol 1977;84:798.
85. Connor CG, Campbell JB, Tirey WW, et al. Modification of impression cytology for in-office use. J Am Optom Assoc 1991;62:898.
86. Hamano H. A new method for measuring tears. Contact Lens Assoc Ophthal J 1983;9:281.
87. Gilbard JP, Farris RL, Samtamaria J. Osmolarity of tear micro-volumes in keratoconjunctivitis sicca. Arch Ophthalmol 1978;96:677.
88. Farris RL, Gilbard JP, Stuchell RN, Mandel ID. Diagnostic tests in keratoconjunctivitis sicca. Contact Lens Assoc Ophthal J 1983;9:23.
89. Mishima J, Gasset A, Klyce CD, Baum JL. Determination of tear volume and tear flow. Invest Ophthalmol 1966;5:264.
90. Lavaux JE, Keller WD. Lacrimal equilibration time (LET): a quick and simple dry eye test. Optom Vis Sci 1993;70:832.
91. Robboy M, Orsborn G. The responses of marginal dry eye lens wearers to a dry eye survey. Contact Lens J 1989;17:8.
92. Golding TR, Efron N, Brennan NA. Soft lens lubricants and prelens tear stability. Optom Vis Sci 1990;67:461.
93. Efron N, Golding TR. The effect of soft lens lubricants on symptoms and lens dehydration. CLAO J 1991;17:114.
94. Aiello JP, Insler MS. The effects of hypotonic and hypertonic solutions on the fluid content of hydrophilic contact lenses. Am J Ophthalmol 1985;99:521.

95. Caffery BE, Josephson JE. Is there a better "comfort drop?" J Am Optom Assoc 1990;61:178.
96. Fatt I, Rocher P. Contact lens performance in different climates. Optom Today (London) 1994;34:26.
97. Korb DR, Greiner JV. Increase in Tear Film Lipid Layer Thickness Following Treatment of Meibomian Gland Dysfunction. In DA Sullivan (ed), Lacrimal Gland, Tear Film, and Dry Eye Syndromes. New York: Plenum, 1994.
98. Ong BL, Larke JR. Meibomian gland dysfunction: some clinical, biochemical and physical observations. Ophthalmic Physiol Opt 1990;10:144.
99. Gutgesell VJ, Stern GA, Hood CI. Histopathology of meibomian gland dysfunction. Am J Ophthalmol 1982;94:383.
100. Caffery BE. Influence of diet on tear function. Optom Vis Sci 1991;68:58.
101. Patel S, Plaskow J, Ferrier C. The influence of vitamins and trace element supplements on the stability of the pre-corneal tear film. Acta Ophthalmol 1993;71:825.
102. Patel S, Ferrier C, Plaskow J. Effect of Systemic Ingestion of Vitamin and Trace Element Dietry Supplements on the Stability of the Pre-Corneal Tear Film in Normal Subjects. In DA Sullivan (ed), Lacrimal Gland, Tear Film, and Dry Eye Syndromes. New York: Plenum, 1994.
103. Brennan NA, Efron N. Hydrogel lens dehydration: a material-dependent phenomenon? Contact Lens Forum 1987;April 28–29, pp 28–29.
104. Brennan NA, Lowe R, Efron N, Harris MG. In vivo dehydration of disposable (Acuvue) contact lenses. Optom Vis Sci 1990;67:201.
105. Mackie IA. Contact lenses in dry eyes. Trans Ophthalmol Soc UK 1985;104:477.
106. Helton DO, Watson LS. Hydrogel contact lens dehydration rates determined by thermogravimetric analysis. CLAO J 1991;17:59.
107. Anderson J, Lowther GE. Dehydration Rates of Selected Hydrogel Lenses. Presented as a poster at the B&L Contact Lens Research Symposium, San Diego, August, 1993.
108. Sorbara L, Talsky C. Contact lens wear in the dry eye patient: predicting success and achieving it. Can J Optom 1988;50:234.
109. Milder B. The Lacrimal Apparatus. In RA Moses, WM Hart (eds), Adler's Physiology of the Eye (8th ed). St. Louis: Mosby, 1987;15.
110. Mathers WD, Daley TE. Evaporation and tear flow in lacrimal insufficiency. Invest Ophthalmol Vis Sci 1994;35:1575.
111. Doane MC. Blinking and the mechanics of the lacrimal drainage system. Ophthalmology 1981;88:844.
112. Lemp MA, Well HH. How do tears exit? Invest Ophthalmol Vis Sci 1983;24:619.
113. Maurice DM. The dynamics and drainage of tears. Int Ophthalmol Clin 1973;13:103.

114. Jones LT, Marquis MM, Vincent NJ. Lacrimal function. Am J Ophthalmol 1972;73:658.
115. von Denffer H, Dressler J, Pabst HW. Lacrimal dacryoscintigraphy. Semin Nucl Med 1984;14:8.
116. Ogut MS, Bavbek T, Kazokoglu H. Assessment of tear drainage by fluorescein dye disappearance test after experimental canalicular obstruction. Acta Ophthalmol 1993;71:69.
117. Meyer DR, Antonello A, Linberg JV. Assessment of tear drainage after canalicular obstruction using fluorescein dye disappearance. Ophthalmology 1990;97:1370.
118. Houlder NA, Forstot SL. Effective duration of intracanalicular collagen implants. Invest Ophthalmol 1994;35:1692.
119. Lowther GE, Semes L. Effect of absorbable intracanalicular collagen implants in hydrogel contact lens patients with drying symptoms. ICLC 1995;22:238.
120. Groves SW, Forstat SL, Lear J. Intracanalicular collagen implants: a dacryoscintigraphic study. Invest Ophthalmol Vis Sci 1991;32:727.
121. Apte RV. Quantitative analysis of tear outflow reduction due to intracanalicular collagen implants using lacrimal scintillography. Invest Ophthalmol Vis Sci 1994;35:1692.
122. Giovagnoli D, Graham SJ. Inferior punctal occlusion with removable punctal plugs in treatment of dry-eye related contact lens discomfort. J Am Optom Assoc 1992;63:481.
123. Norn MS. Tear secretion in diseased eyes. Acta Ophthalmol 1966;44:25.
124. Grohe RM, Caroline PJ. Surface Deposits on Contact Lenses. In ES Bennett, BA Weissman (eds), Clinical Contact Lens Practice. Philadelphia: Lippincott, 1991.
125. Henry VA, Bennett ES, Campbell RC. Explanations for parameter changes on RGP patient lenses. Contact Lens Forum 1989;14(8):57.
126. Boltz KD. The overzealous contact lens cleaner. CL Spectrum 1989;4(12):53.
127. Friedman DM. Too much lens cleaning can also be destructive. Contact Lens Forum 1989;14(9):80.
128. Bennett ES, Henry VA. RGP Lens Power Change with Abrasive Cleaner Use. ICLC 1990;17:152.
129. Lowther GE. Effect of solutions on HGP contact lens parameters. J Am Optom Assoc 1987;58:188.
130. Andrasko G. Peripheral corneal staining: incidence and time course. CL Spectrum 1990;5(7):59.
131. Schnider C. Rigid gas permeable extended wear. CL Spectrum 1990;5:101.
132. Henry VA, Bennett ES, Forrest JM. Clinical investigation of the Paraperm EW rigid gas permeable contact lens. Am J Optom Physiol Opt 1987;64:313.

133. Swarbrick HA, Holden BA. Rigid gas permeable lens binding: significance and conributing factors. Am J Optom Physiol Opt 1987;64:815.
134. Swarbrick HA, Holden BA. Rigid gas-permeable lens adherence: a patient-dependent phenomenon. Optom Vis Sci 1989;66:269.

Index